UN
DI

Sys**tem**atic Reviews

This book
self ser
Fi

Systematic Reviews

Synthesis of Best Evidence for Health Care Decisions

Edited by

Cynthia Mulrow, MD, MSc
Professor of Medicine
Audie L. Murphy Veterans Hospital
San Antonio, Texas

Deborah Cook, MD, MSc(Epid)
Associate Professor of Medicine
St. Joseph's Hospital
Hamilton, Ontario, Canada

American College of Physicians
Philadelphia, Pennsylvania

A|C|P

Manager, Books Program: David Myers
Acquisitions Editor: Mary K. Ruff
Production Supervisor: Allan S. Kleinberg
Production Editor: Karen C. Nolan
Interior and Cover Designer: Barry Moshinski

Composition by Fulcrum Data Services, Inc., Philadelphia, Pennsylvania
Printing/binding by Victor Graphics, Inc., Baltimore, Maryland
Printed in the United States of America

Library of Congress Cataloging-in-Publication Data

Systematic reviews: synthesis of best evidence for health care
  decisions/edited by Cynthia Mulrow and Deborah Cook.
    p. cm.
    Includes bibliographical references and index.
    ISBN 0-943126-66-5 ✓
    1. Systematic reviews (medical research).   I. Mulrow, Cynthia D.
(Cynthia Diane), 1953 .   II. Cook, Deborah, 1960 .
    [DNLM: 1. Review Literature.   2. Research.   3. Meta-Analysis.
4. Decision Support Techniques.   5. Delivery of Health Care.   W
20.5 S995 1998]
R853.S94S95 1998
362.1'07'23—dc21
DNLM/DLC   97-34983
for Library of Congress   CIP

Also Available from the American College of Physicians

SI Units for Clinical Measurement
How to Report Statistics in Medicine

Publications from the BMJ Publishing Group are available to members through
the American College of Physicians.

Customer Service Center
American College of Physicians
Independence Mall West
Sixth Street at Race
Philadelphia, PA 19106-1572
215-351-2600
800-523-1546, ext. 2600

01 02/0 9 8 7 6 5 4 3 2

Contributors

Robert G. Badgett, MD
Assistant Professor of Medicine
University of Texas Health Sciences
     Center at San Antonio
San Antonio, Texas

Lisa A. Bero, PhD
Associate Professor of Medicine
Institute for Health Policy Studies
University of California
     at San Francisco
San Francisco, California

Deborah J. Cook, MD, MSc(Epid)
Associate Professor of Medicine
St. Joseph's Hospital
Hamilton, Ontario, Canada

Carl Counsell, MRCP (UK)
Department of Clinical Neurosciences
Western General Hospital
Edinburgh, Scotland

Frank Davidoff, MD
Editor
Annals of Internal Medicine
American College of Physicians
Philadelphia, Pennsylvania

A. Gray Ellrodt, MD
Division of Internal Medicine
Cedars-Sinai Medical Center
Los Angeles, California

Nancy L. Greengold, MD
Coordinator
Zynx Inc.
Affiliate of Cedars-Sinai Center
Los Angeles, California

Jeremy Grimshaw, MBChB, MRCGP
Health Sciences Research Unit
Department Public Health
Aberdeen, Scotland

R. Brian Haynes, MD, PhD
Professor of Epidemiology and
     Medicine
Health Information Research Unit
Department of Clinical Epidemiology
     and Biostatistics
McMaster University Medical Center
Hamilton, Ontario, Canada

Mark C. Henderson, MD
Program Director of Internal Medicine
University of Texas Health Science
     Center at San Antonio
San Antonio, Texas

Dereck L. Hunt, MD
Postdoctorate Fellow
Health Sciences Center
McMaster University
Hamilton, Ontario, Canada

John P.A. Ioannidis, MD
Therapeutics Research Program
Division of AIDS
National Institute of Allergy
    and Infectious Diseases
Bethesda, Maryland

Alejandro R. Jadad, MD, DPhil
Assistant Professor
Health Information Research Unit
Department of Clinical Epidemiology
    and Biostatistics
McMaster University
Hamilton, Ontario, Canada

Peter Langhorne, PhD, MRCP
Section of Geriatric Medicine
Royal Infirmary
Glasgow, Scotland

Joseph Lau, MD
Division of Clinical Care Research
New England Medical Center
Boston, Massachusetts

K. Ann McKibbon, MLS
Research Librarian
McMaster University Health Sciences
    Center
Hamilton, Ontario, Canada

Henry J. McQuay, DM
Pain Research Unit and Nuffield
    Department of Anaesthetics
Radcliffe Hospital
Oxford, England

Maureen O. Meade, MD, FRCPC, MSc
The Wellesley-Central Hospital
Toronto, Ontario, Canada

R. Andrew Moore, DSc
Pain Research Unit and Nuffield
    Department of Anaestheics
Radcliffe Hospital
Oxford, England

Cynthia D. Mulrow, MD, MSc
Professor of Medicine
Audie L. Murphy Veterans Hospital
San Antonio, Texas

Mary O'Keefe, MD
Assistant Professor of Medicine
University of Texas Health Sciences
    Center at San Antonio
San Antonio, Texas

W. Scott Richardson, MD
Department of Medicine
University of Rochester
School of Medicine and Dentistry
Rochester, New York

Christopher H. Schmid, PhD
Division of Clinical Care Research
New England Medical Center
Boston, Massachusetts

Scott R. Weingarten, MD, MPH
Director
Health Services Research
Cedars-Sinai Medical Center
Los Angeles, California

Contents

Preface

Where is the knowledge we have lost in information?
— *T.S. Eliot, "The Rock"*

Systematic literature reviews, including meta-analyses, are invaluable scientific activities. The rationale for such reviews is grounded firmly in several premises. Firstly, decision makers of various types are inundated with unmanageable amounts of information. Over two million articles are published annually in over 20,000 biomedical journals. Most of us are overwhelmed by this volume and prefer summaries of information to multiple publications of original investigations. Secondly, single studies rarely provide definitive answers to clinical questions. Systematic reviews of multiple studies help establish whether scientific findings are consistent and can be generalized across populations, settings, and treatment variations, or whether findings vary by particular subsets. Thirdly, explicit methods used in systematic reviews limit bias and help improve reliability and accuracy of conclusions. Fourthly, systematic reviews that use quantitative techniques, or meta-analyses, can increase power and precision of estimates of treatment effects and exposure risks. Without systematic reviews, promising leads or small effects can be missed and investigators can embark on studies of questions that have already been answered. Fifthly, systematic reviews identify crucial areas and questions that have not been adequately addressed with past research.

Indeed, the value of systematic reviews is increasingly recognized; their number has multiplied at least 500-fold in the past decade. Guides are available to help critique and apply results from such reviews. New techniques for conducting the reviews have been developed and problems have been identified. For example, methods for formulating questions of systematic reviews are available. Validated approaches for searching electronic bibliographic databases, such as MEDLINE and EMBASE, for various study types, including systematic reviews, are available. New statistical techniques for summarizing data about diagnostic tests and effectiveness of interventions for patient groups with varying baseline risks are evolving. Conceptual and statistical methods for applying results of systematic reviews to individual patients and for helping patients and their health care providers balance benefits and risks of therapies are in their infancy. User-friendly presentation and translation formats for systematic reviews are being tested.

The series of articles published in this book addresses many of the issues described above. The value of systematic reviews for different players, including health care providers, teachers, researchers, and policy-makers, is discussed. Ways to locate, appraise, and use systematic reviews are presented. State-of-the-art methods for conducting systematic reviews are summarized. Moreover, it is our hope that this book will help increase understanding about the important role systematic reviews play in advancing knowledge, facilitate use of systematic reviews, and motivate more reviewers to conduct systematic reviews.

Systematic Reviews: Critical Links in the Great Chain of Evidence

Cynthia D. Mulrow, MD, MSc; Deborah J. Cook, MD, MSc(Epid); and Frank Davidoff, MD

Successful clinical decisions, like most human decisions, are complex (1). In making them, we draw on information from many sources: primary data and patient preferences, our own clinical and personal experience, external rules and constraints, and scientific evidence (Figure). The mix of inputs to clinical decisions varies from moment to moment and from day to day, depending on the decision and the decision makers. In general, however, the proportion of scientific evidence in the mix has grown progressively over the past 150 years or so.

One major reason why the mix has changed is simply the explosive increase in the amount and quality of the scientific evidence that has come from both the laboratory bench and the bedside. The maelstrom of change wrought by the molecular biology revolution has been matched at the clinical level by a tidal wave of increasingly sophisticated clinical trials. It is estimated that since the results of the first randomized clinical trials in medicine were published in the 1940s (2), roughly 100 000 randomized and controlled clinical trials have appeared in print (3), and the results of many well-conducted, completed trials remain unpublished (4). A second reason for the growing emphasis on scientific evidence is the increasing expectation, from both within and outside of the medical profession, that physicians will produce and use "the evidence" in delivering care.

The future holds the promise of continued expansion of the body of research information. However, it also holds the parallel threat of increasingly inadequate time and resources with which to find, evaluate, and incorporate new research knowledge into everyday clinical decision making. Fortunately, mechanisms are emerging that will help us acquire the best, most compelling, and most current research evidence. Particularly promising in this regard is the use of systematic reviews.

Systematic reviews are concise summaries of the best available evidence that address sharply defined clinical questions (5, 6). Of course, the concept of reviews in medicine is not new. Preparation of reviews has traditionally depended on implicit, idiosyncratic methods of data collection and interpretation. In contrast, systematic reviews use explicit and rigorous methods to

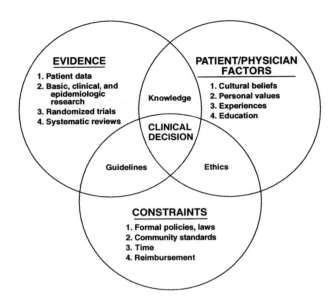

Figure 1. Factors that enter into clinical decisions.

identify, critically appraise, and synthesize relevant studies. As their name implies, systematic reviews—not satisfied with finding part of "the truth"—look for "the whole truth." That is, they seek to assemble and examine all of the available high-quality evidence that bears on the clinical question at hand.

Although it looks easy from the outside, producing a high-quality systematic review is extremely demanding. The realization of how difficult the task is should be reassuring to all of us who have been frustrated by our seeming inability to stay informed and up to date by combing through the literature ourselves. The concepts and techniques involved, including that of meta-analysis, are at least as subtle and complex as many of those currently used in molecular biology. In this connection, it is important to understand that a systematic review and a meta-analysis are not one and the same. Meta-analysis is a specific methodologic and statistical technique for combining quantitative data. As such, it is simply one of the tools—albeit a particularly important

one—that is used in preparing systematic reviews. Although many of the techniques involved in creating a systematic review have been widely available for some time, the techniques for generating clinical recommendations that consider baseline risk, cost, and the totality of the evidence available from a systematic review constitute a relatively new area of research that requires dealing with a range of critical yet abstract issues, such as ambiguity, context, and confidence.

Many articles describing the conceptual basis of systematic reviews have been published during the past decade (7), but detailed, "how-to" information on preparing, understanding, and using systematic reviews has been scattered and incomplete. The following chapters have been designed to collate and update that information. In Chapter 1, Cook and colleagues describe systematic reviews in detail, discuss their strengths and limitations, and explain how they differ from traditional, narrative reviews. The subsequent chapters are divided into two categories: using systematic reviews in practice and conducting systematic reviews.

These chapters are primarily broad narrative overviews. In preparing them, their authors have drawn on widely varying sources, including electronic searches of the published literature, reference lists, the Cochrane Library (3), personal files, colleagues, and personal experience. Most of the chapters are directed toward practitioners who wish to learn more about what systematic reviews are and how to use them. A few are directed primarily toward specific audiences, such as physician-educators. And we hope that the last chapters will entice some readers to join the growing number of groups that are doing the hard but intensely rewarding work of preparing systematic reviews.

Some of the chapters inevitably delve into technical and seemingly arcane methodologic topics, but we make no apologies for this. Medicine at all levels is technical, and "pushing the envelope" inevitably involves moving out into unfamiliar and sometimes uncomfortable territory. Perhaps more important, however, is that many aspects of the systematic review process will be familiar to clinicians because these techniques are similar to the ones they use every day: collecting, filtering, synthesizing, and applying information.

How can the full potential of the knowledge contained in systematic reviews be realized in clinical practice? There is no simple answer, but the following would help. First, developers of electronic databases must, at the very least, pioneer improved—that is, more transparent and clinically meaningful—approaches to searching, thereby giving physicians rapid, sensitive, and specific access to multiple data sources. Second, we need many more systematic reviews that address the natural history and diagnosis of disease and the benefits and potential harms of health care interventions. Third, we need to champion the production of new, well-designed, high-quality research that evaluates important patient outcomes— the "raw material" of systematic reviews that

is a crucial part of clinical decision making. And, finally, both physicians and the health care systems in which we work need to fully embrace and tangibly support lifelong learning as an essential element in the practice of good medicine.

A recent related development is an international movement to improve the reporting of clinical research, particularly the results of randomized, controlled trials (9) and meta-analyses (10). These efforts focus on clear, comprehensive communication of the methods and results of clinically relevant research through the development and application of reporting standards that are being suggested by editors, researchers, methodologists, and consumers. These standards should allow readers to better appraise, interpret, and apply the information in published reports of research in their own practices and situations. Perhaps equally important is the possibility that these standards will create a positive "ripple effect," starting at the earliest stages of research planning and extending through the conduct of clinical trials.

Exciting new information pouring out of the molecular biology revolution has the potential to transform medicine. But even this enormously powerful information will be of little use to physicians and their patients unless 1) the diagnostic and therapeutic interventions that flow from it are stringently tested in clinical trials and 2) the results of those trials are synthesized and made accessible to practitioners. Systematic reviews are thus a vital link in the great chain of evidence that stretches from the laboratory bench to the bedside. From this perspective, the awesome task of extracting the knowledge already encoded in the tens of thousands of high-quality clinical studies, published and unpublished, is arguably every bit as important to our health and well-being as the molecular biology enterprise itself. The task can only grow in size and importance as more and better trials are conducted; indeed, the task has already been likened in scope and importance to the Human Genome Project (11).

It is our earnest hope that this collection of systematic reviews will play a useful part in strengthening the chain of evidence that links research to practice.

References

1. **Damasio AR.** Descartes' Error: Emotion, Reason, and the Human Brain. New York: GP Putnam; 1994.
2. **Hart PD.** Early controlled clinical trials [Letter]. BMJ. 1996;312:378-9.
3. The Cochrane Collaboration. The Cochrane Library. Oxford, United Kingdom: Update Software; 1996 [updated quarterly].
4. **Bero L, Rennie D.** The Cochrane Collaboration. Preparing, maintaining, and disseminating systematic reviews of the effects of health care. JAMA. 1995;274:1935-8.
5. **Mulrow CD.** The medical review article: state of the science. Ann Intern Med. 1987;106:485-8.
6. **Mulrow CD.** Rationale for systematic reviews. In: Chalmers I, Altman DG, eds. Systematic Reviews. London: BMJ; 1995:1-8.
7. **Chalmers I, Altman DG, eds.** Systematic Reviews. London: BMJ; 1995.
8. **Cook DJ, Mulrow CD, Haynes RB.** Systematic reviews: synthesis of best evidence for clinical decisions. Ann Intern Med. 1997;126:376-80.
9. **Begg C, Cho M, Eastwood S, Horton R, Moher D, Olkin I, et al.** Improving the quality of reporting of randomized controlled trials. The CONSORT statement. JAMA. 1996;276:637-9.
10. **Moher D, Olkin I.** Meta-analysis of randomized controlled trials. A concern for standards. JAMA. 1995;274:1962-3.
11. **Naylor CD.** Grey zones of clinical practice: some limits to evidence-based medicine. Lancet. 1995;345:840-2.

Chapter 1

Synthesis of Best Evidence for Clinical Decisions

Deborah J. Cook, MD, MSc(Epid); Cynthia D. Mulrow, MD, MSc; and R. Brian Haynes, MD, PhD

Systematic reviews can help practitioners keep abreast of the medical literature by summarizing large bodies of evidence and helping to explain differences among studies on the same question. A systematic review involves the application of scientific strategies, in ways that limit bias, to the assembly, critical appraisal, and synthesis of all relevant studies that address a specific clinical question. A meta-analysis is a type of systematic review that uses statistical methods to combine and summarize the results of several primary studies. Because the review process itself (like any other type of research) is subject to bias, a useful review requires clear reporting of information obtained using rigorous methods. Used increasingly to inform medical decision making, plan future research agendas, and establish clinical policy, systematic reviews may strengthen the link between best research evidence and optimal health care.

At the end of a long week in the office, you sink back into your chair, reflecting on some of the more memorable patients you cared for and counseled. Through gentle history taking, you discovered that urinary incontinence is the underlying cause of an elderly patient's increasing social isolation. During a careful physical examination, you detected bruising on the torso of a woman with chronic headaches and began to explore the long-standing abusive relationship between the woman and her alcoholic partner. You discontinued procainamide therapy in a 72-year-old man who had asymptomatic premature ventricular contractions after myocardial infarction. To prevent bleeding from esophageal varices, you started β-blocker therapy in a woman with long-standing cryptogenic cirrhosis and portal hypertension. In couples' therapy, discussing the future quality of life of a middle-aged gay man with human immunodeficiency virus infection, you journeyed through emotionally intense dialogue about advance directives. You presented the risk factors for major and minor bleeding to a 39-year-old woman who was considering warfarin therapy because of recently diagnosed atrial fibrillation and valvular heart disease. You listened to, made diagnoses for, treated, advised, and comforted many patients.

Yet there were some hiccoughs in your practice along the way. You stumbled while debating the pros and cons of breast cancer screening with a healthy 48-year-old woman who has been staying current with information on the Internet. You questioned the merits of a personalized walking program suggested to you by a motivated 66-year-old man with severe claudication. Explaining that you wanted to review the best current evidence on these issues, you resolved to address your uncertainties before these patients made their next office visits, in a week's time.

Sighing deeply, you acknowledge that you have little time to read. You subscribe to three journals, which you browse months after they arrive—either when your journal stack becomes precariously high or when your guilt is sufficiently motivational. You sometimes find the conclusions of individual articles conflicting or confusing. You know that some of the decisions and suggestions you made this week, specifically your decisions about stopping procainamide therapy and starting β-blocker therapy and your advice about bleeding risks from anticoagulant therapy, were based on the best current research evidence (1-3). On the other hand, your patients' inquiries about breast cancer screening and exercise treatment for claudication highlight your need for a concise, current, rigorous synthesis of the best available evidence on each of these topics: in brief, a systematic review (4, 5).

Incorporating Research Evidence into Clinical Decision Making

The foregoing scenario is familiar to practitioners. In a typical week, we encounter patients with diverse problems; exercise numerous clinical, interpersonal, and technical skills; and make many decisions. The factors that affect these decisions and their outcomes are complex. For instance, each patient has unique sociodemographic characteristics, cultural circumstances, and personal preferences. Each physician has unique knowledge, experiences, and values. Moreover, practitioners and their patients make decisions within the context of a rapidly changing health care system that influences the availability, accessibility, and cost of diagnostic tests and therapies (6).

Timely, useful evidence from the biomedical literature should be an integral component of clinical decision making. If one treatment has been shown to be better than another, we need to know, so that we can recommend the treatment to the appropriate patients. The worldwide effort to develop new tests and treatments, and to determine their usefulness, has never been stronger, and our patients and their families expect us to be fonts of the knowledge that results from this effort (7). Unfortunately, it is easy for current best research evidence to pass us by (8). We may lack the time, motivation, and basic skills needed to find, critically appraise, and synthesize information, all of which we must do if we are to integrate the results of original studies into our practice. Fortunately, several potent methods are emerging that can greatly enhance our ability to interpret and apply research evidence; foremost among them is the systematic review.

Systematic reviews represent the best chance that most practitioners will have to understand and accurately apply the key signals arising from the robust and increasingly productive search for solutions to medical problems. A properly conducted systematic review faithfully summarizes the evidence from all relevant studies on the topic of interest, and it does so concisely and transparently.

What Is a Systematic Review?

Systematic reviews are scientific investigations in themselves, with pre-planned methods and an assembly of original studies as their "subjects." They synthesize the results of multiple primary investigations by using strategies that limit bias and random error (9, 10). These strategies include a comprehensive search of all potentially relevant articles and the use of explicit, reproducible criteria in the selection of articles for review. Primary research designs and study characteristics are appraised, data are synthesized, and results are interpreted.

When the results of primary studies are summarized but not statistically combined, the review may be called a qualitative systematic review. A quantitative systematic review, or meta-analysis, is a systematic review that uses statistical methods to combine the results of two or more studies. The term "overview" is sometimes used to denote a systematic review, whether quantitative or qualitative. Summaries of research that lack explicit descriptions of systematic methods are often called narrative reviews.

Review articles are one type of integrative publication; practice guidelines, economic evaluations, and clinical decision analyses are others. These other types of integrative articles often incorporate the results of systematic reviews. For example, practice guidelines are systematically developed statements intended to assist practitioners and patients with decisions about appropriate health care for specific clinical circumstances (11). Evidence-based practice guidelines are based on systematic reviews of the literature, appropriately adapted to local circumstances and values. Economic evaluations compare both the costs and the consequences of different courses of action; the knowledge of consequences that are considered in these evaluations is often generated by systematic reviews of primary studies. Decision analyses quantify both the likelihood and the valuation of the expected outcomes associated with competing alternatives.

Differences Between Systematic and Narrative Reviews

All reviews, narrative and systematic alike, are retrospective, observational research studies and are therefore subject to systematic and random error. Accordingly, the quality of a review—and thus its worth—depends on the extent to which scientific review methods have been used to minimize error and bias. This is the key feature that distinguishes traditional narrative reviews from systematic reviews (Table 1.1). If a review is prepared according to the steps outlined in the right column of Table 1.1, it is more likely to be systematic and to provide unbiased conclusions. If review methods approximate those found in the middle column of Table 1.1, the article is more likely to be a narrative review, and the conclusions are less likely to be based on an unbiased summary of all relevant evidence.

Systematic reviews are generated to answer specific, often narrow, clinical questions in depth. These questions can be formulated explicitly according to four variables: a specific population and setting (such as elderly outpatients), the condition

Table 1.1   Differences between Narrative Reviews and Systematic Reviews

Feature	Narrative Review	Systematic Review
Question	Often broad in scope	Often a focused clinical question
Sources and search	Not usually specified, potentially biased	Comprehensive sources and explicit search strategy
Selection	Not usually specified, potentially biased	Criterion-based selection, uniformly applied
Appraisal	Variable	Rigorous critical appraisal
Synthesis	Often a qualitative summary	Quantitative summary*
Inferences	Sometimes evidence-based	Usually evidence-based

*A quantitative summary that includes a statistical synthesis is a meta-analysis.

of interest (for example, hypertension), an exposure to a test or treatment (such as pharmacologic management), and one or more specific outcomes (such as cardiovascular and cerebrovascular events and mortality) (12). Thus, an example of a well-formulated, clinically relevant question is, Does pharmacologic treatment of hypertension in the elderly prevent strokes and myocardial infarctions or delay death? If the question that is driving the review is not clear from the title, abstract, or introduction, or if no methods section is included, the paper is more likely to be a narrative review than a systematic review (13).

Most narrative review articles deal with a broad range of issues related to a given topic rather than addressing a particular issue in depth (9). For example, a narrative review on diabetes (such as that which might be found in a textbook chapter) might include sections on the physiology and pathophysiology of carbohydrate, lipid, and protein metabolism; the epidemiology of and prognosis associated with diabetes; diagnostic and screening approaches; and preventive, therapeutic, rehabilitative, and palliative interventions. Thus, narrative reviews may be most useful for obtaining a broad perspective on a topic; they are less often useful in furnishing quantitative answers to specific clinical questions.

Narrative reviews are appropriate for describing the history or development of a problem and its management. Narrative reviews may better describe cutting-edge developments if research is scant or preliminary or if studies are very limited by flawed design or execution (13). They may be particularly useful for discussing data in light of underlying theory and context. Narrative reviews can draw analogies and can conceptually integrate two independent fields of research, such as cancer and the acquired immunodeficiency syndrome (13).

However, the connection between clinical recommendations and evidence in narrative reviews is often tenuous, incomplete, or—worse still—based on a biased citation of studies (14, 15). As a result, recommendations found in narrative reviews published in journals and textbooks often differ from recommendations found in systematic reviews. For example, narrative reviews may lag behind by more than a decade in endorsing a treatment of proven effectiveness, or they may continue to advocate a therapy long after it has been shown to be useless or harmful (16). Also, systematic reviews that incorporate quantitative techniques are more likely than narrative reviews to detect small but clinically meaningful treatment effects (17).

What Systematic Reviews Can and Cannot Do

A well-conducted systematic review is invaluable for practitioners. Many of us feel overwhelmed by the volume of medical literature and, as a result, often prefer summaries of information to publications of original investigations (18). Thus, review articles can help us keep up to date. High-quality systematic reviews can define the boundaries of what is known and what is not known and can help us avoid knowing less than has been proven.

It is unusual for single studies to provide definitive answers to clinical questions (19), but systematic reviews can help practitioners solve specific clinical problems. By critically examining primary studies, systematic reviews can also improve our understanding of inconsistencies among diverse pieces of research evidence. By quantitatively combining the results of several small studies, meta-analyses can create more precise, powerful, and convincing conclusions. An example of this is the recent review highlighting the beneficial effect of dietary protein restriction on the progression of diabetic and nondiabetic renal disease (20). In addition, systematic reviews of several studies may better inform us about whether findings can be applied to specific subgroups of patients (21).

Investigators need systematic reviews to summarize existing data, refine hypotheses, estimate sample sizes, and help define future research agendas. Without systematic reviews, researchers may miss promising leads or may embark on studies of questions that have been already answered. Administrators and purchasers need review articles and other integrative publications to help generate clinical policies that optimize outcomes using available resources (22).

Systematic reviews can aid, but can never replace, sound clinical reasoning. Clinicians reason about individual patients on the basis of analogy, experience, heuristics, and theory as well as research evidence (23-25). Awareness of a treatment's effectiveness does not confer knowledge about how to use that treatment in caring for individual patients. Evidence can lead to bad practice if it is applied in an uncritical or unfeeling way (25). Understanding the complex structure of medical decision making (26) requires an appreciation of the ways in which knowledge, skills, values, and research evidence are integrated in each patient-clinician encounter.

The Past, Present, and Future of Systematic Reviews

The epidemiology of review articles is changing rapidly; the number of systematic reviews published annually has increased at least 500-fold in the past decade (27, 28). It is not unusual now to find more than one systematic review addressing the same or similar therapeutic questions (29). One example is the evaluation of the effect of calcium on blood pressure, which was summarized in two recent meta-analyses published within 1 month of each other

(30, 31). Although duplicate independent reviews that generate similar results may increase our confidence in those results, multiple reviews with similar results may have an opportunity cost—they may divert effort away from the development of systematic reviews in other areas where they may be needed. The situation can become more confusing when several reviews yield similar results but present different clinical recommendations; this occurred when five meta-analyses of selective decontamination of the digestive tract in critically ill patients were published within 5 years (two were published in the same issue of the same journal) (32-36). However, resolving discord between meta-analyses can be a cooperative, informative exercise that clarifies review methods and synthesizes all currently available evidence (37).

In the past 10 years, guides have been created to aid in the critical appraisal (38, 39) and application (40) of review articles. A framework for interpreting primary research and systematic reviews by using levels of evidence and grades of recommendations (41) has been successfully employed by several groups. At the Antithrombotic Consensus Conferences of the American College of Chest Physicians, therapeutic recommendations are routinely classified according to their evidentiary base—whether they are predicated on the results of large, rigorous, randomized trials or on meta-analyses, observational studies, or expert opinion (41).

An international initiative called the *Cochrane Collaboration* has evolved to help prepare, maintain, and disseminate the results of systematic reviews of health care interventions (42, 43). The Cochrane Library is the first large-scale, multidisciplinary product of this collaboration. It is updated quarterly, and in January 1997 it contained 159 completed systematic reviews and 199 systematic reviews in preparation from the Cochrane Collaboration itself, a bibliography of more than 1600 other systematic review abstracts in the medical literature, a register of controlled trials that included slightly more than 110 000 trials, and a bibliography of 400 methodologic articles about the science of reviewing research (44).

What does the future hold for systematic reviews? The coverage of medical topics by systematic reviews, although expanding rapidly, is still limited. The Cochrane Collaboration is facilitating this mission but needs increasing support and participation if it is to succeed. Investigation into the science of research synthesis will increase the quality, and thus the value, of the evidence found in systematic reviews. More efficient searching methods with which to identify systematic reviews will be developed. Patients and administrators will have increasing access to reviews, which will spur practitioners to locate, appraise, and apply reviews in their practice.

Information technology can provide point-of-care access, but practitioners will need new skills to use such technology. Presentation formats will become more user-friendly for both providers and patients. Practical techniques for incorporating information from systematic reviews into clinical decision making will be created and disseminated.

While looking forward to these advances, clinicians can and should take advantage of what systematic reviews have to offer now. *Systematic Reviews* will aid in that process by focusing on how to find, assess, use, and conduct systematic reviews for clinical, teaching, and research purposes.

Key Points To Remember

- Systematic reviews assemble, critically appraise, and synthesize the results of primary investigations addressing a specific topic or problem.
- Systematic reviews are prepared using strategies that limit bias and random error.
- Systematic reviews are integrative articles; other examples of integrative articles are economic evaluations, practice guidelines, and clinical decision analyses.
- Systematic reviews can help practitioners keep up to date with the overwhelming volume of medical literature.
- Systematic reviews can help ground clinical decisions in research evidence, although they neither make decisions nor obviate the need for sound, compassionate clinical reasoning.

Acknowledgments: We would like to acknowledge many persons for their advice and support:

Advisors: Gordon Guyatt (Hamilton, Ontario, Canada), R. Brian Haynes (Hamilton, Ontario, Canada), Andrew Oxman (Oslo, Norway), and David L. Sackett (Oxford, England).

Reviewer-Commentators: Iain Chalmers (Oxford, England), Robert Fletcher (Boston, Massachusetts), Larry V. Hedges (Chicago, Illinoïs), Andreas Laupacis (Ottawa, Ontario, Canada), C. David Naylor (North York, Ontario, Canada), and David L. Simel (Durham, North Carolina).

Clinical Reviewers: Clifton R. Cleaveland (Chattanooga, Tennessee), Paul F. Speckart (San Diego, California), and Norman J. Wilder (Anchorage, Alaska).

Local Editorial Assistants: Linn Morgan and Barbara Hill.

Grant Support: Dr. Cook is a Career Scientist of the Ontario Ministry of Health; Dr. Mulrow is Senior Research Associate at the Audie L. Murphy Memorial Veterans Hospital; and Dr. Haynes is a National Health Scientist of the National Health Research and Development Program of Health Canada.

References

1. **Teo KK, Yusuf S, Furberg CD.** Effects of prophylactic antiarrhythmic drug therapy in acute myocardial infarction. An overview of results from randomized controlled trials. JAMA. 1993; 270:1589-95.
2. **Pagliaro L, D'Amico G, Sorensen TI, Lebrec D, Burroughs AK, Morabito A, et al.** Pre-

vention of first bleeding in cirrhosis. A meta-analysis of randomized trials of nonsurgical treatment. Ann Intern Med. 1992;117:59-70.

3. **Landefeld CS, Beyth RJ.** Anticoagulant-related bleeding: clinical epidemiology, prediction, and prevention. Am J Med. 1993;95:315-28.

4. **Kerlikowske K, Grady D, Rubin SM, Sandrock C, Ernster VL.** Efficacy of screening mammography. A meta-analysis. JAMA. 1995;273: 149-54.

5. **Gardner AW, Poehlman ET.** Exercise rehabilitation programs for the treatment of claudication pain. A meta-analysis. JAMA. 1995;274:975-80.

6. **Sackett DL, Haynes RB.** On the need for evidence-based medicine. Evidence-Based Medicine. 1995;1:5-6.

7. **Evidence-Based Medicine Working Group.** Evidence-based medicine. A new approach to teaching the practice of medicine. JAMA. 1992;268:2420-5.

8. **Shin JH, Haynes RB, Johnston ME.** The effect of problem-based, self-directed undergraduate education on life-long learning. Can Med Assoc J. 1993;148:969-76.

9. **Mulrow CD.** The medical review article: state of the science. Ann Intern Med. 1987;106:485-88.

10. **Cook DJ, Sackett DL, Spitzer WO.** Methodologic guidelines for systematic reviews of randomized control trials in health care from the Potsdam Consultation on Meta-Analysis. J Clin Epidemiol. 1995;48:167-71.

11. **Woolf SH.** Practice guidelines: a new reality in medicine. I. Recent developments. Arch Intern Med. 1990;150:1811-8.

12. **Richardson WS, Wilson MC, Nishikawa J, Hayward RS.** The well-built clinical question: a key to evidence-based decisions [Editorial]. ACP J Club. 1995;123:A12.

13. **Bangert-Drowns RL.** Misunderstanding meta-analysis. Evaluation and the Health Professional. 1995;18:304-14.

14. **Ravnskov U.** Cholesterol lowering trials in coronary heart disease: frequency of citation and outcome. BMJ. 1992;305:15-9.

15. **Neihouse PF, Priske SC.** Quotation accuracy in review articles. DICP. 1989;23:594-6.

16. **Antman EM, Lau J, Kupelnick B, Mosteller F, Chalmers TC.** A comparison of results of meta-analyses of randomized control trials and recommendations of clinical experts. Treatments for myocardial infarction. JAMA. 1992;268:240-8.

17. **Cooper HM, Rosenthal R.** Statistical versus traditional procedures for summarizing research findings. Psychol Bull. 1980;87:442-9.

18. **Williamson JW, German PS, Weiss R, Skinner EA, Bowes F 3d.** Health science information management and continuing education of physicians. A survey of U.S. primary care practitioners and their opinion leaders. Ann Intern Med. 1989;110:151-60.

19. **Davidoff F.** Evidence-based medicine: why all the fuss? [Editorial] Ann Intern Med. 1995;122:727.

20. **Pedrini MT, Levey AS, Lau J, Chalmers TC, Wang PH.** The effect of dietary protein restriction on the progression of diabetic and nondiabetic renal diseases: a meta-analysis. Ann Intern Med. 1996;124:627-32.

21. **Antiplatelet Trialists' Collaboration.** Collaborative overview of randomised trials of antiplatelet therapy-I: Prevention of death, myocardial infarction, and stroke by prolonged antiplatelet therapy in various categories of patients. BMJ. 1994;308:81-106.

22. **Milne R, Hicks N.** Evidence-based purchasing. Evidence-Based Medicine. 1996;1:101-2.

23. **Tanenbaum SJ.** What physicians know. N Engl J Med. 1993;329:1268-71.

24. **McDonald CJ.** Medical heuristics: the silent adjudicators of clinical practice. Ann Intern Med. 1996;124(1 Pt 1):56-62.

25. **Naylor CD.** Grey zones of clinical practice: some limits to evidence-based medicine. Lancet. 1995;345:840-2.

26. **Dowie J.** "Evidence-based", "cost-effective" and "preference-driven" medicine: decision analysis-based medical decision making is the pre-requisite. Journal of Health Services Research and Policy. 1996;1:104-13.

27. **Chalmers TC, Lau J.** Meta-analytic stimulus for changes in clinical trials. Stat Methods Med Res. 1993;2:161-72.

28. **Chalmers I, Haynes RB.** Reporting, updating, and correcting systematic reviews of the effects of health care. In: Chalmers I, Altman DG, eds. Systematic reviews. London: BMJ; 1995:86-95.

29. **Jadad A, Cook DJ, Browman G.** When arbitrators disagree: resolving discordant meta-analysis. Can Med Assoc J. 1997; [In press].

30. **Allender PS, Cutler JA, Follmann D, Cappuccio FP, Pryer J, Elliott P.** Dietary calcium and blood pressure: a meta-analysis of randomized clinical trials. Ann Intern Med. 1996;124:825-31.

31. **Bucher HC, Cook RJ, Guyatt GH, Lang JD, Cook DJ, Hatala R, Hunt DL.** Effects of dietary calcium supplementation on blood pressure. A meta-analysis of randomized controlled trials. JAMA. 1996;275:1016-22.

32. **Vandenbroucke-Grauls CM, Vandenbroucke JP.** Effect of selective decontamination of the digestive tract on respiratory tract infections and mortality in the intensive care unit. Lancet. 1991;338:859-62.

33. **Hurley JC.** Prophylaxis with enteral antibiotics in ventilated patients: selective decontamination or selective cross-infection? Antimicrobial Agents Chemother. 1995;39:941-7.

34. **Selective Decontamination of the Digestive Tract Trialists' Collaborative Group.** Meta-analysis of randomized controlled trials of selective decontamination of the digestive tract. Br Med J. 1993;307:525-32.

35. **Heyland DK, Cook DJ, Jaeschke R, Griffith L, Lee HN, Guyatt GH.** Selective decontamination

of the digestive tract. An overview. Chest. 1994;105:1221-9.

36. **Kollef MH.** The role of selective digestive tract decontamination on mortality and respiratory infections. A meta-analysis. Chest. 1994;105:1101-8.

37. **Cook DJ, Reeve BK, Guyatt GH, Griffith LE, Heyland DK, Buckingham L, et al.** Stress ulcer prophylaxis in critically ill patients. Resolving discordant meta-analyses. JAMA. 1996;275:308-14.

38. **L'Abbe KA, Detsky AS, O'Rourke K.** Meta-analysis in clinical research. Ann Intern Med. 1987;107:224-33.

39. **Oxman AD, Cook DJ, Guyatt GH.** Users' guides to the medical literature. VI. How to use an overview. Evidence-Based Medicine Working Group. JAMA. 1994;272:1367-71.

40. **Guyatt GH, Sackett DL, Sinclair J, Hayward R, Cook DJ, Cook RJ.** Users' guides to the medical literature. IX. A method for grading health care recommendations. Evidence-Based Medicine Working Group. JAMA. 1995;274:1800-4.

41. **Cook DJ, Guyatt GH, Laupacis A, Sackett DL, Goldberg RJ.** Clinical recommendations using levels of evidence for antithrombotic agents. Chest. 1995;108(4 Suppl):227S-30S.

42. **Chalmers I.** The Cochrane Collaboration: preparing, maintaining, and disseminating systematic reviews of the effects of health care. Ann N Y Acad Sci. 1993;703:153-63.

43. **Bero L, Rennie D.** The Cochrane Collaboration. Preparing, maintaining, and disseminating systematic reviews of the effects of health care. JAMA. 1995;274:1935-8.

44. **Cochrane Collaboration.** Cochrane Library. Electronic serial publication issued quarterly by BMJ Publishing Group, London.

Chapter 2

Locating and Appraising Systematic Reviews

Dereck L. Hunt, MD; and K. Ann McKibbon, MLS

We describe the strengths and weaknesses of several methods of locating systematic reviews, including electronic databases such as MEDLINE, Best Evidence (the electronic version of *ACP Journal Club* and *Evidence-Based Medicine*), and the Cochrane Library (a regularly updated source of reviews and controlled trials produced by the Cochrane Collaboration). We also present steps that can be used to critically appraise review articles; as an example, we use a systematic review that evaluates the gastrointestinal toxicity of various nonsteroidal anti-inflammatory drugs in the context of a clinical scenario.

This chapter has two purposes: to describe tools and techniques that can help locate systematic reviews effectively and efficiently, and to suggest a method of critically appraising the methodologic quality of these reviews. The latter is a necessary step in determining whether the results of a systematic review should be used in practice and, if so, how they should be used.

Clinical Scenario

Your patient is a 65-year-old man who has painful osteoarthritis in both knees and no other major medical conditions. Although he can still carry out his activities of daily living, he has limited mobility and reports pain at rest. You are now reviewing his history and current care with him. You had previously prescribed acetaminophen, 4 g/d, which provided minimal pain relief. The patient is eager to try a different medication. You mention that nonsteroidal anti-inflammatory drugs (NSAIDs) are generally not associated with improved analgesia compared with acetaminophen (1), but the patient still wants to try an alternate medication. You agree to offer him short-term NSAID therapy but are not sure which agent has the lowest rate of serious gastrointestinal complications, such as hemorrhage. You suspect that many original studies have been published that discuss the risks of different NSAIDs, but you would like to have a succinct and accurate summary of the study results rather than having to do all of the searching, selecting, and synthesizing yourself. Because this question is important to your patient and common in your practice, you proceed to look for a systematic review.

Locating Systematic Reviews

Internists have several valuable sources of systematic reviews: MEDLINE and other electronic databases, journals, Best Evidence (the electronic version of *ACP Journal Club* and *Evidence-Based Medicine*), and the Cochrane Library. Each resource has advantages and disadvantages.

Electronic Databases

The largest and most readily available tool for locating systematic reviews is MEDLINE, a multipurpose database produced by the U.S. National Library of Medicine. In MEDLINE and related databases, the National Library of Medicine indexes important biomedical literature from more than 4000 journals. The MEDLINE database has more than 7 000 000 citations that date back to 1966; 5 000 000 of these citations deal with humans. One tenth of the citations are indexed as review articles, but only a small fraction of these review articles are systematic reviews.

Because of the size and complexity of MEDLINE, searching this database for systematic reviews requires careful planning and an understanding of the terms and phrases used to describe systematic reviews (which form the basis of your search strategy). They include the adjectives "quantitative," "methodological," and "systematic" to describe either "reviews" or "overviews." Another phrase, less commonly used, is "review articles with a methods section." "Meta-analysis" has been spelled in various ways (meta-analysis, metaanalysis, metaanalyses, meta-analyses, meta analysis, meta analyses).

To facilitate searching, you need to be aware of how indexers classify and index systematic reviews and meta-analyses. The indexers at the National Library of Medicine recognize meta-analyses and index them using the Medical Subject Heading (MeSH) "meta-analysis (MeSH)" and the publication type (pt) "meta-analysis (pt)." They do not, however, recognize systematic reviews as different from traditional review articles. All review articles (systematic or otherwise) are indexed with the publication type "review (pt)." One way to identify the systematic reviews is to limit review articles to those that include the term "MEDLINE" in their abstract. To do so, the search terms "review (pt) AND MEDLINE (textword)" are used. "MEDLINE" is included here because most clinical systematic reviews include a description of how the component original studies were identified and because the term "MEDLINE" is often included in the abstract.

By using the preceding list of terms and phrases, we can create a search strategy to identify systematic reviews that are indexed in MEDLINE. Most MEDLINE access systems allow search strategies to be stored for easier searching in the future. Research efforts by members of the Cochrane Collaboration are currently under way to establish the most sensitive and specific search strategies for locating systematic reviews for questions about therapy. These strategies will complement those that have been developed to locate primary studies on therapy, diagnosis, cause, and prognosis (2). Until this work has been completed, the following two search strategies (one simple approach and one more complex approach) are useful. The second strategy identifies many of the systematic reviews that are indexed in MEDLINE.

The simple search consists of the following steps:

1. meta-analysis (pt)
2. meta-anal: (textword) [see the appendix for explanation of the symbol ":" and other MEDLINE searching functions]
3. review (pt) AND medline (textword)

1 OR 2 OR 3

The comprehensive search consists of the following steps:

1. meta-analysis (pt)
2. meta-anal: (textword)
3. metaanal: (textword)
4. quantitativ: review: OR quantitative: overview: (textword)
5. systematic: review: OR systematic: overview: (textword)
6. methodologic: review: OR methodologic: overview: (textword)
7. review (pt) AND medline (textword)

1 OR 2 OR 3 OR 4 OR 5 OR 6 OR 7

Next, content terms are added to narrow the search to our clinical topic. For this search, we need to include terms for NSAIDs, adverse effects, and gastrointestinal complications. Articles on NSAIDs are indexed under the MeSH term "anti-inflammatory agents, non-steroidal"; this term is used for the family of drugs and for individual drugs. The National Library of Medicine recognizes 38 NSAIDs, from aminopyrine to tolmetin. We want to search on any NSAID, so we ask MEDLINE to "explode" the phrase. We then specify that these drugs must be the main topic of the article (this is done by "starring" or "majoring," depending on the search system you use). We only want articles that look at side effects (adverse effects) of the NSAIDs, and thus we stipulate this criterion. We then use the "AND" command to cross this search for articles on NSAIDs with the search for systematic reviews. This combined search strategy yields seven citations, published in English from 1992 to the present; two seem to be exactly on the topic of interest (3, 4). The other five address mucosal protective agents, economics, effects of NSAIDs on blood pressure, methodologic issues, and a case report that includes a review of the literature.

After retrieving the two potentially relevant articles, we find that the paper by Carson and Willett (4) examines the toxic effects of NSAIDs as a group, whereas the paper by Henry and colleagues (3) addresses our clinical question of which NSAID is associated with the fewest gastrointestinal side effects.

The European "MEDLINE" is EMBASE, the electronic version of *Excerpta Medica.* This database has a strong European content and little overlap with MEDLINE in terms of the journals covered. New publications are included more quickly in EMBASE than in MEDLINE. The EMBASE database places special emphasis on physical and occupational therapy, biology, drug research, psychiatry, health policy, and alternative medicine. The database is produced in the Netherlands by Elsevier, a commercial company. User costs are higher than those for MEDLINE, and few clinicians outside Europe have ready access to it. Librarians, however, can often provide EMBASE searches.

The EMBASE search for our scenario (done using a strategy and content terms similar to those used in the comprehensive MEDLINE search) retrieved 30 citations and cost $60. Several citations were unique and interesting, but none appeared to address our question any better than those that we had already identified through MEDLINE.

Journals

Most major medical journals publish systematic reviews. Using the comprehensive MEDLINE search strategy described earlier, we identified 117 citations in *Annals of Internal Medicine* from 1992 to June 1996 that may represent systematic reviews. In the same period, *JAMA* published 106 reviews, *BMJ* published 97, *Archives of Internal Medicine* published 40, and *The New England Journal of Medicine* published 21. Because so few systematic reviews are published in each issue, journals are not necessarily a high-yield source of systematic reviews for clinical problem solving. However, finding systematic reviews while browsing through journals can obviously help keep clinicians up to date.

Best Evidence

A new resource called Best Evidence, produced by the American College of Physicians, can be used to efficiently identify systematic reviews on clinical topics of interest to internists. Best Evidence is the electronic version of both *ACP Journal Club* and *Evidence-Based Medicine*. These publications contain structured abstracts of and expert commentary on high-quality, clinically important studies from more than 75 medical journals (5). Each article must meet certain minimum methodologic quality standards. For example, studies on therapy must have used random allocation to the comparison groups, have had at least 80% follow-up, and have measured a clinically important outcome. This means that articles on therapy abstracted in Best Evidence are likely to be valid and relevant to patient care (6, 7). To be included in Best Evidence, review articles must address a specific clinical question and describe how potentially relevant primary studies were identified and either included or excluded. All review articles in Best Evidence (approximately 10% to 20% of the current total of more than 1000 articles) are systematic reviews rather than narrative reviews. Most of them contain the term "meta-analysis" or "review" in their short title.

Returning to our initial scenario, we search Best Evidence using the terms "NSAID" and "gastrointestinal" and retrieve nine citations. Two are systematic reviews that look potentially useful; one of the two is the review by Henry and colleagues (3). Best Evidence is easy to use, but it may not include a systematic review if it was recently published or was not published in the journals that are scanned for *ACP Journal Club* and *Evidence-Based Medicine*.

Cochrane Library

A quick way to identify systematic reviews for therapeutic issues is to use the Cochrane Library, produced by the Cochrane Collaboration (8, 9). The diskette and CD-ROM versions of the Cochrane Library are updated quarterly, and an Internet version is currently being developed. The Library has four sections: the Cochrane Database of Systematic Reviews, the Database of Abstracts of Reviews of Effectiveness (DARE), the Cochrane Controlled Trials Registry, and the Cochrane Review Methodology Database.

These systematic reviews cover many areas of health care (including consumer concerns) and are often more thorough reports of systematic reviews that have been published elsewhere in limited form. The Cochrane Database of Systematic Reviews and DARE are the sections of the Library that are most useful to clinicians interested in identifying systematic reviews. Version 3 of the Cochrane Database of Systematic Reviews (updated in November 1996) contains 141 systematic reviews that were done under the auspices of the Collaboration. In addition, the authors of the reviews are committed to updating the reviews as new information becomes available. The reviews include listings of excluded trials and the reasons for exclusion, information that most traditional systematic reviews do not report. Produced by the National Health Services Centre for Reviews and Dissemination (located at the University of York, United Kingdom), DARE contains citations to 1422 non-Cochrane systematic reviews along with structured abstracts of many of the reviews.

To address the question raised by the patient in our scenario, we search the November 1996 Cochrane Library by using the term "nonsteroidal." This identifies one protocol in the Cochrane Database of Systematic Reviews and six systematic reviews in DARE. One systematic review seems potentially relevant to our question but is different from the two identified by the MEDLINE search.

The Cochrane Library is a quick and valuable resource for locating systematic reviews, but it has some limitations. The first is its modest size; however, the number of reviews is increasing as more systematic reviews are published. The second limitation is that searching can be difficult, especially when complex search strategies are used. This area, however, will be improved in future releases. The third limitation is that few clinicians have access to the Cochrane Library. Increasing subscriptions and the Internet version (http://www.medlib.com) will help to rectify this situation.

Assessing the Quality of a Systematic Review

The article by Henry and colleagues (3) may answer our question about which NSAID is associated with the fewest serious gastrointestinal complications. However, the strength of inference we can draw from the review depends on the review methods used. Assessment of the validity of a review requires evaluation of each step in the review process before consideration of the results and how they might apply to our patient.

Oxman and colleagues (10) have proposed one set of simple criteria for evaluating systematic reviews that builds on criteria published in a validated index for the assessment of the quality of review articles (11, 12). This index includes questions on the reporting of the adequacy of search methods, comprehensiveness of the search, inclusion criteria, assessment of selection bias, documentation and appropriateness of the validity criteria used, reporting of methods used to combine study results, appropriateness of pooling of studies, the extent to which the report's conclusions were supported by the data, and a global assessment of scientific quality. In the following analysis, we consider eight major determinants of the quality of the review and examine how they apply to the systematic review by Henry and colleagues (3).

1. *Did the review address a focused question?* Henry and colleagues did not examine all complications associated with NSAID use in any setting. They did, however, define their research question—to evaluate different NSAIDs and focus on the association between these drugs and peptic ulcer complications that required hospitalization.

2. *Is it likely that important, relevant studies were missed?* Our confidence in the results of a review is greater when we are certain that no relevant and high-quality studies, either published or unpublished, were missed. A comprehensive search for unpublished work may be important in some situations (for example, evaluation of new technologies, an area in which much of the data may not be published) if the data are amenable to the same careful assessment of quality as the published work. Resource constraints may also limit search strategies. Assessing the comprehensiveness of the search obviously requires that the authors of reviews explicitly report their methods.

Henry and colleagues used a CD-ROM system to search MEDLINE for articles published between 1985 and 1994, but they did not describe their exact search strategy. They also examined the bibliographies of two published reviews and contacted authors of relevant studies, asking them to identify additional research. Although Henry and colleagues could have searched additional databases such as EMBASE or hand-searched selected journals, their approach was reasonable.

3. *Were the inclusion criteria used to select articles appropriate?* These criteria may vary according to the population studied, interventions or exposures, outcomes,

and methods of each study. Henry and colleagues clearly stated that cohort and case-control studies were selected if the patients had been living in the community, had been taking NSAIDs, and had been hospitalized for gastrointestinal hemorrhage or perforation. They stated which studies were included and why; they also presented their rationale and made their list of excluded trials available upon request.

4. *Was the validity of the included studies assessed?* Although the conclusions we derive from a systematic review depend in large part on the rigor of the review methods, they obviously also depend on the quality of the included studies. The appropriate criteria for this assessment of quality depend on the type of studies included in the review (10). For example, if the systematic review deals with treatment, it is important to ascertain whether the trials were randomized; whether the randomization process was concealed from patients or investigators; whether patients, caregivers, or persons assessing outcome were blinded to the treatment allocation; and the extent to which follow-up was complete. For systematic reviews that address questions of harm, the most important considerations include documentation of the similarity of the comparison groups and the methods used to establish that patients had the exposure and outcome of interest (13). Duration of follow-up is also important if a cohort design was used.

In their article on the relative risk for gastrointestinal complications with different NSAIDs, Henry and colleagues state that they evaluated each of the factors mentioned in the preceding paragraph but did not report them in the article. The summary tables, however, are available on request from the authors.

5. *Were the assessments of studies reproducible?* Even when explicit criteria are used to include studies in a review and evaluate their methodologic quality, the

judgment of the review's authors is still required. If the authors did each of the review steps independently and in duplicate and then reported their level of agreement, we can assess how open to judgment each of these steps was. Agreement beyond that expected by chance is often reported using the κ statistic (14), which ranges from 0 to 1. The closer the value is to 1, the greater the level of agreement. Henry and colleagues reported that they extracted data in duplicate and resolved differences by consensus. They did not assess the eligibility or quality of the articles in duplicate.

6. *Were the results similar from study to study?* Synthesizing the results of studies (whether qualitative or quantitative) requires assessing the similarity of the studies to each other. This means that the patients, exposures or interventions, outcomes, and other features of study design must be considered. Pooling the results of several studies is not appropriate if the studies differ in a clinically important fashion with regard to any of these design elements. If, on the other hand, all the studies appear similar after this initial assessment, it is then important to evaluate whether the results of the studies were similar. If studies have different findings, pooling results may lead to meaningless or even misleading results. Such variability in results often suggests that the trials may have differed in some important way, more than initially seemed to be the case; the sources of the differences then become the appropriate focus of interest.

How can we determine whether the results of trials included in a meta-analysis are similar? The size of the treatment effect (and its CI) from each trial can be graphed. If the magnitude or direction of the effect sizes differs greatly among studies and if the CIs do not substantially overlap, one could question whether it is appropriate to pool the results.

Another common approach is to use a statistical test to ascertain whether the study results differ more than would be expected by chance. If the studies measure approximately the same effect and any differences occur because of chance (that is, if the results are consistent with a common effect size), the test for homogeneity (sometimes, unfortunately, called the test of heterogeneity) is not significant (usually reported as P ">" 0.05). A significant test result means that the difference in results among the individual studies is not likely to have been caused by chance. This calls into question whether it is appropriate to pool the results; it may also suggest that *a priori* subgroup analyses may be appropriate. However, when the results of large trials are pooled, the test for homogeneity may indicate that statistically significant (but perhaps clinically unimportant) differences exist in the results. In this situation, it may still be reasonable to pool the results statistically.

Henry and colleagues established that the results of their included studies were consistent. They calculated the risk for gastrointestinal complications associated with each NSAID relative to the risk associated with ibuprofen and then tested whether the relative risk for each drug was consistent across the studies. Table 2.1, originally published in the systematic review by Henry and colleagues, shows the relative risk, CIs, and P values for each of these tests for consistency (homogeneity). Each P value is greater than 0.05.

7. *What are the overall results and how precise are they?* We have considered the key methodologic questions to be asked when appraising a review article and believe that the methods used by Henry and colleagues are satisfactory. Because another chapter in this volume will focus on measures of effect, we only briefly address this issue here.

Henry and colleagues identified 12 studies that were relevant and met their inclusion criteria. They then abstracted the data in duplicate, calculated the relative risks associated with each NSAID, and pooled the relative risk estimates. They found that each NSAID was associated with a higher risk for gastrointestinal complications than was ibuprofen and ranked the drugs in order of increasing size of risk (ranging from 1.6 for fenoprofen to 9.2 for azapropazone). The authors also calculated CIs around the pooled estimates. All NSAIDs except fenoprofen were associated with an increased risk for serious gastrointestinal hemorrhage compared with ibuprofen.

8. *Will the results help in caring for patients?* Determining this involves asking several questions: Can I apply the results to my patients? Did the studies consider all the clinically important outcomes? Are the benefits worth any associated risks or costs?

It is important to consider the patients in the individual studies and to ascertain whether your patient is similar with regard to age, comorbid conditions, or other risk factors (such as smoking and family history). Does he or she have a comparable baseline risk for the outcome of interest, or is the risk higher or lower in a clinically meaningful way? A systematic review that finds that a new treatment delays death but that does not address any of the potential adverse events associated with use of the treatment may prompt us to seek additional information from other sources or to refer back to some of the more detailed original articles. We would want to discuss these issues with our patient (or we may choose not to offer the intervention in the first place).

We decide that the review by Henry and colleagues is rigorous, the results are convincing, and the patient in our clinical scenario is similar to the study patients (all of whom were living in a community setting before hospitalization). Because this patient with severe osteoarthritis insists on trying a medication other than acetaminophen, you prescribe ibuprofen on the

Table 2.1   Risk for Gastrointestinal Complications in Patients Receiving Nonsteroidal Anti-Inflammatory Drugs*

Nonsteroidal Anti-Inflammatory Drug	Studies, *n*	Relative Risk (95% CI)	*P* Value
Ibuprofen	—	1.0	—
Fenoprofen	2	1.6 (1.0–2.5)	0.31
Aspirin	6	1.6 (1.3–2.0)	0.69
Diclofenac	8	1.8 (1.4–2.3)	0.78
Sulindac	5	2.1 (1.6–2.7)	0.69
Diflunisal	2	2.2 (1.2–4.1)	0.35
Naproxen	10	2.2 (1.7–2.9)	0.13
Indomethacin	11	2.4 (1.9–3.1)	0.49
Tolmetin	2	3.0 (1.8–4.9)	0.30
Piroxicam	10	3.8 (2.7–5.2)	0.09
Ketoprofen	7	4.2 (2.7–6.4)	0.26
Azapropazone	2	9.2 (4.0–21.)	0.83

*Adapted from Henry and colleagues (3) with permission of BMJ.

basis of the systematic review and then follow him to assess his response.

Summary

Several methods can be used to identify systematic reviews. These include bibliographic databases, such as MEDLINE, Best Evidence, and the Cochrane Library. In the future, the Cochrane Library could become the source of choice for systematic reviews because it provides the full text of Cochrane reviews and citations to many other systematic reviews. Moreover, the Library is growing rapidly and becoming more readily available, and its searching capabilities are being improved with each update. Although Best Evidence contains fewer systematic reviews than the Cochrane Library, it is specifically designed for practicing internists and primary care physicians and includes systematic reviews on diagnosis, cause, prognosis, and quality improvement. At present, however, MEDLINE and other bibliographic databases are probably the most up to date and readily available sources of systematic reviews.

Systematic reviews are a powerful and useful way to assemble evidence; however,

just because a review has been done using systematic review methods does not guarantee that its results are credible. Regardless of the source, all systematic reviews (like all types of research evidence) require critical appraisal to determine their validity and to establish whether and how they will be useful in practice.

Key Points To Remember

• MEDLINE and other electronic databases, Best Evidence, and the Cochrane Library are useful sources of systematic reviews.

• Because the Cochrane Library includes only systematic reviews, searching terms can be limited to content terms.

• To use MEDLINE efficiently in locating systematic reviews, specifically tailored searching strategies are necessary.

• A comprehensive approach to evaluating systematic reviews is important before their results are applied.

• Steps in the critical appraisal process include assessing the exhaustiveness of the search, selection criteria, quality of the included studies, and whether study designs and results are similar across studies.

Appendix:
Terminology and Strategies
for MEDLINE Searches

MEDLINE searching uses many concepts and terms. To facilitate optimal use of MEDLINE, several of the most important are described below. The examples are drawn from the search for systematic reviews on NSAIDs and gastrointestinal complications.

Indexing

All citations in MEDLINE are indexed for content and methods using the MeSH vocabulary, which consists of 14 000 specific terms and 18 000 synonyms. Two aspects of MEDLINE indexing are particularly worth keeping in mind. First, terminology is not always intuitive, so the vocabulary should be checked in a printed or electronic compendium of MeSH terms. Second, all articles are indexed according to the most specific MeSH heading or headings available. In other words, if you wanted to find an article specifically about ibuprofen, you would not find it by simply looking under the parent MeSH heading "anti-inflammatory agents, non-steroidal."

Major Subject Headings (Starring or Majoring)

Many articles deal predominantly with one or two topics and briefly mention several other subjects (usually 5 to 15). When articles are indexed, they are assigned MeSH terms for each topic referred to in the paper. To make searching more powerful and selective, MeSH terms that indicate the major focus or emphasis of the paper are specially coded. Some MEDLINE searching systems do this by placing an asterisk (*) before the MeSH heading, hence the term "starring." Other systems simply refer to these as major aspects of the article ("majoring").

Exploding

"Exploding" refers to a MEDLINE search technique that enables users to circumvent the fact that all articles are indexed using the most specific MeSH heading available. It also allows the user to gather similar MeSH terms together. Using the term "exploding" instructs MEDLINE to identify all articles that have been indexed using a broad "family" MeSH term itself (for example, gastrointestinal diseases), as well as all articles indexed by more specific MeSH terms that are listed in the MeSH hierarchy under the broad term. To use the NSAID example again, a MEDLINE search that uses the MeSH term "anti-inflammatory agents, non-steroidal" would identify only articles that deal with NSAIDs in general. If, on the other hand, "explode" was used along with "anti-inflammatory agents, non-steroidal," all articles on any of the 38 specific NSAIDs and those on NSAIDs in general would be identified.

Textwords

If you are searching for an article on a subject that has not been well indexed using MeSH terms, it is often helpful to have MEDLINE search the text of the titles and abstracts in the database for certain "free text" words or phrases. Our search strategy for systematic reviews illustrates this point. Systematic reviews are not indexed in MEDLINE. Thus, to identify them, our strategy largely relies on textword searching using the various free terms for systematic reviews that authors have used in their titles and abstracts. The search strategy for systematic reviews also illustrates another feature of textword searching. If you are unsure of the final letters that an author may have used at the end of a word, you can insert a symbol such as ":" (the symbol varies from system to system). For example, the instruction "random:" tells MEDLINE to search for the words "random," "randomized," "randomization," "randomised," "randomisation," and "randomly."

Acknowledgments: The authors thank the clinical reviewer, Clifton R. Cleveland, and R. Brian Haynes, Alex Jadad, and Andreas Laupacis for thoughtful reviews of the manuscript.

Grant Support: Health Evidence Application Linkage Network Research Fellowship (Dr. Hunt).

References

1. **Bradley JD, Brandt KD, Katz BP, Kalasinski LA, Ryan SI.** Comparison of an antiinflammatory dose of ibuprofen, an analgesic dose of ibuprofen, and acetominophen in the treatment of patients with osteoarthritis of the knee. N Engl J Med. 1991;325:87-91.

2. **Haynes RB, Wilczynski N, McKibbon KA, Walker CJ, Sinclair JC.** Developing optimal search strategies for detecting clinically sound studies in MEDLINE. J Am Med Inform Assoc. 1994;1:447-58.

3. **Henry D, Lim LL, Garcia Rodriguez LA, Perez Gutthann S, Carson JL, Griffin M, et al.** Variablility in risk of gastrointestinal complications with individual non-steroidal anti-inflammatory drugs: results of a collaborative meta-analysis. BMJ. 1996;312:1563-6.

4. **Carson J, Willett LR.** Toxicity of nonsteroidal anti-inflammatory drugs. An overview of the epidemiological evidence. Drugs. 1993;46(Suppl 1):243-8.

5. **Haynes RB.** Selection of articles for ACP Journal Club according to content [Editorial]. ACP J Club. 1992;117:A18-9.

6. **Guyatt GH, Sackett DL, Cook DJ.** Users' guides to the medical literature. II. How to use an article about therapy or prevention. A. Are the results of the study valid? Evidence-Based Medicine Working Group. JAMA. 1993;270:2598-601.

7. **Guyatt GH, Sackett DL, Cook DJ.** Users' guides to the medical literature. II. How to use an article about therapy or prevention. B. What were the results and will they help me in caring for my patients? Evidence-Based Medicine Working Group. JAMA. 1994;271:59-63.

8. **Bero L, Rennie D.** The Cochrane Collaboration. Preparing, maintaining, and disseminating systematic reviews on the effects of health care. JAMA. 1995;274:1935-8.

9. **Huston P.** Cochrane Collaboration helping unravel the tangled web woven by international research. Can Med Assoc J. 1996;154:1389-92.

10. **Oxman AD, Cook DJ, Guyatt GH.** Users' guides to the medical literature. VI. How to use an overview. Evidence-Based Medicine Working Group. JAMA. 1994;272:1367-71.

11. **Oxman AD, Guyatt GH, Singer J, Goldsmith CH, Hutchison BG, Milner RA, et al.** Agreement among reviewers of review articles. J Clin Epidemiol. 1991;44:91-8.

12. **Oxman AD, Guyatt GH.** Validation of an index of the quality of review articles. J Clin Epidemiol. 1991;44:1271-8.

13. **Levine M, Walter S, Lee H, Haines T, Holbrook A, Moyer V.** Users' guides to the medical literature. IV. How to use an article about harm. Evidence-Based Medicine Working Group. JAMA. 1994;271:1615-9.

14. **Landis JR, Koch GG.** The measurement of observer agreement for categorical data. Biometrics. 1977;33:159-74.

Chapter 3

Using Numerical Results from Systematic Reviews in Clinical Practice

Henry J. McQuay, DM; and R. Andrew Moore, DSc

Systematic reviews summarize large amounts of information and are more likely than individual trials to describe the true clinical effect of an intervention. Traditional statistical outputs from meta-analyses cannot immediately be applied to clinical practice. The number needed to treat (NNT) has that clinical immediacy. This number can be calculated easily from raw data or from statistical outputs, and the principle involved in its calculation can be applied to different outcomes: treatment efficacy, adverse events (harm), or other dicotomous end points. The NNT defines the treatment-specific effect of an intervention, and we suggest it as a tool for making decisions about individual patients. Knowing the NNT for different interventions that have the same outcome for the same disorder can help shape individual and institutional practice. Estimating the number needed to harm is also an important part of the equation. Estimating an individual patient's baseline risk can, with the NNT, be a guide to the overall or net value of a prophylactic or therapeutic intervention. NNTs from meta-analyses or individual randomized trials are simple to remember and directly support efforts to work with patients to make the best possible clinical decisions for their care.

As professionals, we want to use the best treatments; as patients, we want to be given them. Knowing whether an intervention works (or does not work) is fundamental to clinical decision making. However, clinical decision making involves more than simply taking published results of research directly to the bedside. Physicians need to consider how similar their patients are to those in the published studies, to take the values and preferences of their patients into account, and to consider their own experience with a given test or treatment.

Evidence from clinical research is becoming increasingly important in medical-practice decisions as more and better evidence is published. But when is the evidence strong enough to justify changing a practice? Individual studies that involve only small numbers of patients may have results that are distorted by the random play of chance and thus lead to less than optimal decisions. As is clear from other chapters in this book, systematic reviews identify, critically appraise, and review all the relevant studies on a clinical question and are more likely to give a valid answer. They use explicit methods and quality standards to reduce bias. Their results are the closest we can come to reaching the truth given our current state of knowledge.

The questions about an intervention that a systematic review should answer are the following:

1. Does it work?
2. If it works, how well does it work in general and compared with placebo, no treatment, or other interventions that are currently in use?
3. Is it safe?
4. Will it be safe and effective for my patients?

Whereas the critical appraisal and qualitative synthesis provided by review articles can be interpreted directly, the numerical products of quantitative reviews can be more difficult to understand and apply in daily clinical practice. This chapter provides guidance on how to interpret the statistical results of systematic reviews, translate these results into more understandable terms, and apply them directly to individual patients. Many of these principles can also be used to interpret the numerical results of individual clinical studies. They are particularly relevant to systematic reviews, however, which often exert greater influence than do individual studies.

Making Sense of the Numerical Results of Clinical Studies

Although the results of clinical studies can be expressed in intuitively meaningful ways, such results do not always easily translate into clinical decision making. For example, results are frequently expressed in terms of *risk*, which is an expression of the frequency of a given outcome. (Risks are probabilities, which can vary between 0.0 and 1.0. A probability of 0.0 means that the event will never happen, and a probability of 1.0 means that it always happens.)

Consider a hypothetical study of the recurrence of migraine headaches in a control group receiving placebo and a treatment group receiving a new antimigraine preparation, drug M (a secondary prevention trial). Suppose that at the end of the trial, migraines recurred in 30% of the control group (the risk for recurrence was 0.30) but in only 5% of the drug M group (risk of 0.05) (Table 3.1).

The outcomes of the study are clear enough for the two groups when they are examined separately. But clinicians and patients are more interested in the comparative results, that is, the outcome in one group relative to the outcome in the other group. This overall (comparative) result can be expressed in various ways. For example, the *relative risk*, which is the risk in the treatment group relative to that in the control group, is simply the ratio of the risks in the two groups. In other words, relative risk is the risk in the treatment group divided by that in the control group, $0.05 \div 0.30$, or 0.17. The comparison can also be expressed as the *reduction in relative risk*, which is the ratio between the decrease in risk (in the treatment group) and the risk in the control group, $0.25 \div 0.30$, or 0.83 (Table 3.1). (The relative risk reduction can also be calculated as 1 − relative risk.)

Although the clinical meaning of relative risk (and relative risk reduction) is reasonably clear, relative risk has the distinct disadvantage that a given value (for example, 0.17) is the same whether the risk with treatment decreases from 0.80 to 0.14, from 0.30 to 0.05, from 0.001 to 0.00017, and so forth. The clinical implications of these changes clearly differ from one another enormously and depend on the specific disease and intervention. An important alter-

Table 3.1   Numerical Expression of Hypothetical Clinical Trial Results

Variable	Trial of Drug M for Migraine		Trial B		Trial C	
	Treatment Group	Control Group	Treatment Group	Control Group	Treatment Group	Control Group
Group size, n	100	100				
Recurrences, n	5	30				
Risk for recurrence*	0.05 (*a*)	0.30 (*b*)	0.14 (*a*)	0.8 (*b*)	0.00017 (*a*)	0.001 (*b*)
Relative risk: *a/b*	0.17 (*c*)		0.17 (*c*)		0.17 (*c*)	
Relative risk reduction: (*b* − *a*)/*b* or 1 − *c*	0.83 (*d*)		0.83 (*d*)		0.83 (*d*)	
Absolute risk reduction: *b* − *a*	0.25 (*e*)		0.66 (*e*)		0.00083 (*e*)	
Number needed to treat: 1/*e*	4		1.5		1204	
Odds	0.053 (*f*)	0.43 (*g*)				
Odds ratio: *f/g*	0.12					

*Can also be expressed as a percentage (% risk = risk × 100).

nate expression of comparative results, therefore, is the *absolute risk reduction.* Absolute risk reduction is determined by subtracting the risk in one group from the risk in the other (for example, the risk in the treatment group is subtracted from the risk in the placebo group). In the case of our migraine study, the absolute risk reduction would be 0.30 − 0.05, which equals 0.25, or 25 percentage points. In contrast, for a study in which the risk decreased from 0.001 to 0.00017, the absolute risk reduction would be only 0.00083, or 0.083 percentage points, which is a trivial change in comparison (Table 3.1).

This arithmetic emphasizes the difficulty of expressing the results of clinical studies in meaningful ways. Relative risk and relative risk reduction clearly give a quantitative sense of the effects of an intervention in proportional terms but provide no clue about the size of an effect on an absolute scale. In contrast, although it tells less about proportional effects, absolute risk says a great deal about whether an effect is likely to be clinically meaningful. Despite this benefit, even absolute risk is problematic because it is a dimensionless, abstract num-

ber; that is, it lacks a direct connection with the clinical situation in which the patient and physician exist. However, another way of expressing clinical research results can provide that clinical link: the *number needed to treat* (NNT).

Number Needed To Treat

The NNT for a given therapy is simply the reciprocal of the absolute risk reduction for that treatment (1, 2). In the case of our hypothetical migraine study (in which risk decreased from 0.30 without treatment with drug M to 0.05 with treatment with drug M, for a relative risk of 0.17, a relative risk reduction of 0.83, and an absolute risk reduction of 0.25), the NNT would be 1 ÷ 0.25, or 4. In concrete clinical terms, an NNT of 4 means that you would need to treat approximately four patients with drug M to prevent migraine from recurring in one patient. To emphasize the difference between the concepts embodied in NNT and relative risk, recall the various situations mentioned above, in all of which the relative risk was 0.17 but in which the absolute risk decreased from 0.80 to 0.14 in one case and from 0.001 to 0.00017 in another. Note that the corresponding NNTs in these two other cases are 1.5 and 1204, respectively: that is, you would need to treat 1.5 and 1204 patients to obtain a therapeutic result in these two situations compared with 4 patients with drug M (Table 3.1).

The NNT can be calculated easily and kept as a single numerical reminder of the effectiveness (or, as we will see, the potential for harm) of a particular therapy when the outcome is binary or dichotomous. As we suggested, the NNT has the advantage of applicability to clinical practice because it suggests the effort that is required to achieve a particular target. The NNT has the additional advantage that it can be applied to any beneficial outcome or any adverse event (when it becomes the number needed to harm [NNH]). The concept of NNT always refers to a comparison group (in which patients receive placebo, no treatment, or some other treatment), a particular treatment outcome, and a defined period of treatment. In other words, the NNT is the number of patients that you will need to treat with drug or treatment A to achieve an improvement in outcome compared with drug or treatment B for a treatment period of C weeks (or other unit of time). To be fully specified, NNT and NNH must always specify the comparator, the therapeutic outcome, and the duration of treatment that is necessary to achieve the outcome.

Important Qualities of the Number Needed To Treat

The NNT is treatment specific. It describes the difference between treatment and control in achieving a particular clinical outcome. Table 3.2 shows NNTs from a selection of systematic reviews and large randomized, controlled trials.

A very small NNT (that is, one that approaches 1) means that a favorable outcome occurs in nearly every patient who receives the treatment and in few patients in a comparison group. Although NNTs close to 1 are theoretically possible, they are almost never found in practice. However, small NNTs do occur in some therapeutic trials, such as those comparing antibiotics with placebo in the eradication of *Helicobacter pylori* infection or those examining the use of insecticide for head lice (Table 3.2). An NNT of 2 or 3 indicates that a treatment is quite effective. In contrast, such prophylactic interventions as adding aspirin to streptokinase to reduce 5-week vascular mortality rates after myocardial infarction may have NNTs as high as 20 to 40 and still be considered clinically effective.

Limitations of the Number Needed To Treat

Although NNTs are powerful instruments for interpreting clinical effects, they also have important limitations. First, an NNT is generally expressed as a single number, which is known as its point estimate. As with all experimental measurements, however, the true value of the NNT can be higher or lower than the point estimate determined through clinical studies. The 95% CIs of the NNT are useful in this regard because they provide an indication that, 19 times out of 20, the true value of the NNT falls within the specified range. An NNT with a wide CI may include the possibility of no benefit or harm. Such a point estimate may still have clinical importance as a benchmark until further data permit the determination of a finite CI, but clinical decisions must take this large degree of uncertainty into account.

Second, it is inappropriate to compare NNTs across disease conditions, particularly when the outcomes of interest differ. For example, an NNT of 30 for preventing deep venous thrombosis may be valued differently from an NNT of 30 for preventing a disabling stroke or for preventing death.

The concept expressed by the NNT is thus one of frequency, not of utility; its numerical value is a function of the disease, the intervention, and the outcome. If we have NNTs for different interventions for the same condition (and severity) with the same outcome, then, and only then, is it appropriate to directly compare NNTs.

Third, NNTs are not fixed quantities. The NNT for a specified intervention in an individual patient depends not only on the nature of the treatment but also on the risk at baseline (that is, the probability at baseline that the patient being considered will experience the outcome of interest). Because that risk may not be the same for all patients, an NNT that is provided by the literature may have to be adjusted to compensate for your patient's risk at baseline, as described below. Moreover, the concept of NNT assumes that a given intervention produces the same relative risk reduction whether the patient's risk at baseline is low, intermediate, or high. This assumption may not always hold because, for example, a disease may be more difficult to treat when it is severe than when it is mild.

Finally, an NNT is always based on an outcome for a specified period. Imagine a disease that is treated by one injection or by regular daily tablets; the NNTs for the two treatments cannot be directly compared. Only when the outcome is the same and is measured during the same period is a comparison valid.

How Should Numbers Needed To Treat Derived from Systematic Reviews Be Used?

The distinction between therapy and prophylaxis is not always clear (for example, drugs for the treatment of hypertension). Because NNTs may be used differently in the two circumstances, however, it is often useful to distinguish therapy from prophylaxis. Thus, in situations that call for therapeutic intervention (treatment), some

form of therapy will almost always be used, and the key issue therefore is the relative effectiveness of different interventions. For prophylaxis we more often have the choice of doing nothing; the issue then becomes a decision of whether doing something to prevent a bad outcome will be more successful than doing nothing. In contrast, in the case of treatment, the therapeutic equation for most patients consists of weighing the risks and benefits for each of the possible treatments. Under most circumstances, the equation for prophylaxis also includes the possibility of harm without benefit for a considerable number of the patients. For simplicity, therefore, we will separate treatment and prophylaxis and take a few examples from each.

Treatment

The NNT is particularly useful for treatments if several treatments are assessed for the same outcome measure in patients with similar conditions. Using the NNTs, we can rank these treatments relative to one another; this ranking is particularly helpful in making a choice on the basis of effectiveness. However, the resulting NNT league tables are not decision-making aids themselves because NNTs need to be balanced against adverse events; costs; and patient characteristics, expectations, and preferences. It is also important to keep in mind that favorable outcomes can occur without treatment and that the frequency at which this happens affects the NNT.

An example of the relative ranking of treatments can be seen in a comparison of studies of subcutaneous sumatriptan compared with placebo (NNT, 2.0) and oral sumatriptan compared with placebo (NNT, 2.6) for the relief (at 2 hours) of migraine headaches (Table 3.2). Because subcutaneous sumatriptan is more expensive than oral sumatriptan and the NNTs for the two treatments are similar, patient preference may be the deciding factor in choosing

Table 3.2   Numbers Needed To Treat from Systematic Reviews and Randomized, Controlled Trials

Topic of Study (Reference)	Intervention	Duration of Intervention	Comparator	Outcome	Odds Ratio (95% CI)	Number Needed To Treat (95% CI)
Treatment						
Head lice (4)	Permethrin	14 days	Placebo	Cure		1.1 (1.0–1.2)*
Peptic ulcer (5)	Triple therapy	6–10 weeks	Histamine antagonist	Eradication of *Helicobacter pylori*	44 (34–56)	1.1 (1.08–1.15)
Peptic ulcer (5)	Triple therapy	6–10 weeks	Histamine antagonist	Ulcers remaining cured at 1 year	9.4 (6.3–14.0)	1.8 (1.6–2.1)
Migraine (6)	Subcutaneous sumatriptan	One dose	Placebo	Headache relieved at 2 hours		2.0 (1.8–2.2)*
Migraine (6)	Oral sumatriptan	One dose	Placebo	Headache relieved at 2 hours		2.6 (2.3–3.2)*
Fungal nail infection (7)	Terbinafine	12 or 24 weeks	Griseofulvin	Cured at 48 weeks	4.5 (2.3–8.8)	2.7 (1.9–4.5)*
Moderate or severe postoperative pain (8)	Acetaminophen, 1000 mg	One dose	Placebo	Pain relief ≥50%		3.6 (3.0–4.4)
Esophageal variceal bleeding (9)	Endoscopic ligation	Intervention	Sclerotherapy	Prevention of one additional episode of bleeding		4
Peptic ulcer (5)	Triple therapy	6–10 weeks	Histamine antagonist	Ulcer healing at 6–10 weeks compared with histamine antagonist	5.0 (3.3–7.7)	4.9 (4.0–6.4)
Acute otitis media (10)	Antibiotics	Short course	No antibiotics or tympanocentesis	Absence of presenting signs and symptoms at 7–14 days	2.9 (1.8–4.1)	7
Peripheral artery disease (11)	Naftidrofuryl	3 or 6 months	Placebo	Pain-free walking distance improved by 50% at 1 year	1.5 (1.2–2.0)	10.3 (6.3–29)*
Childhood depression (12)	Antidepressants	Not stated	Placebo	Improvement	1.1 (0.5–2.2)	Not effective
Prophylaxis						
Postoperative vomiting (13)	Droperidol	One dose	Placebo	Prevention for 48 hours in children undergoing squint correction	2.5 (1.7–3.6)	4.4 (3.1–7.1)
Venous thromboembolism (14)	Graduated compression stockings	Not stated	No stockings	Episodes of venous thromboembolism	0.3 (0.2–0.4)	9 (7–13)*
Anticipated preterm delivery (15)	Corticosteroids	Before delivery	No treatment	Risk for fetal respiratory distress syndrome		11 (8–16)*
Dog bite (16)	Antibiotics	Short course	Placebo	Infection	0.6 (0.4–0.8)	16 (9–92)*
Hypertension in the elderly (17)	Drug treatments	≥1 year	No treatment	Overall prevention of cardiovascular event for 5 years		18 (14–25)

Continued.

Table 3.2   Numbers Needed To Treat from Systematic Reviews and Randomized, Controlled Trials—
            Continued

Topic of Study (Reference)	Intervention	Duration of Intervention	Comparator	Outcome	Odds Ratio (95% CI)	Number Needed To Treat (95% CI)
Myocardial infarction (18)	Aspirin plus streptokinase	1-hour intra-venous infusion of streptokinase and 1 month of oral aspirin	No treatment	Prevention of one 5-week vascular death		20*
Peripheral artery disease (11)	Naftidrofuryl	3 or 6 months	Placebo	Prevention of critical cardiac events at 1 year compared with placebo	0.6 (0.4–0.96)	24 (13–266)*
Major gastro-intestinal bleeding and use of non-steroidal anti-inflammatory drugs (19)	Misoprostol	6 months	Placebo	Prevention of any gastrointestinal complication	0.6 (0.4–0.85)	166 (97–578)*
Herpes zoster (20)	Acyclovir	5–10 days	Placebo	Prevention of post-hepatic neuralgia at 6 months	0.7 (0.5–1.1)	Not effective

*Calculated from data in the report.

between formulations. An appropriate prescription for a woman in her mid-30s who has relatively frequent headaches and a high-powered position that involves a considerable amount of travel might be subcutaneous sumatriptan, but a retired biochemist who is troubled only by an occasional migraine might be more comfortable with oral sumatriptan. Knowledge about relative effectiveness can be accumulated as additional evidence appears, often from large randomized, controlled trials. If several studies show that aspirin plus metoclopramide for migraine had an NNT of 3 (21), for example, patients and clinicians might elect to change to this alternate therapy because of its lower cost and similar effectiveness when compared with the other two.

Another example of NNT ranking can be seen in reviews of treatments of diabetic neuropathy. Painful diabetic neuropathy affects about 3% of all diabetic patients after 20 years with diabetes. Four systematic reviews of drug treatments have used different approaches (Table 3.3).

The NNTs for antidepressant agents as a class (NNT, 2.5) were similar to those for anticonvulsant agents as a class (NNT, 2.9) in diabetic neuropathy (Table 3.3), but these systematic reviews do not tell us which individual drug was best in either class. Moreover, although the NNT for capsaicin was higher (NNT, 4.2), the overlap of the CIs for the NNTs of all three treatments suggests that we do not have definitive information with which to decide whether capsaicin is the least effective. We may, however, be prepared to make a judgment about whether the effectiveness as determined by the physician (the outcome measure used in the studies of capsaicin) is better or worse than pain relief of more than 50% as judged by the patient (the outcome measure used for the other two drug classes) (Table 3.2). Physician judgments are less sensitive than patient scoring (26). For minor and major harm, no data were available on capsaicin. For minor harm (adverse effects) and major harm (withdrawal from the study because of drug-related toxicity), however, we know that anticonvulsant agents and antidepressant agents carry the same risk.

Choice of treatment for an individual patient depends on several issues. For example, this choice may be determined primarily by whether any of these drugs is licensed for the treatment of diabetic neuropathy (an external rule or constraint), by familiarity with a particular drug (physician knowledge and experience), by patient idiosyncrasy (patient factors), and so on. The point is that systematic reviews can provide valuable information that helps patient and physician to know with reasonable assurance what to expect from treatment.

Prophylaxis

With prophylaxis, the issue is the risk for an event occurring without prophylaxis compared with the risk with prophylaxis. Whether the medical condition is of major public health importance, such as heart attack or stroke, or less threatening, such as animal bites and the risk for subsequent infection, more people at risk will actually be unaffected than affected. The NNTs for prophylaxis tell us about the effectiveness for a population but are more difficult to use when deciding how to manage an individual patient.

As is the case for therapeutic interventions, part of the process of using information from systematic reviews of prophylax-

Table 3.3   Summary of Four Systematic Reviews of Drug Treatments for Painful Diabetic Neuropathy

Variable	Onghena and Van Houdenhove (22)*	Zhang and Li Wan Po (23)	McQuay et al. (24)	McQuay et al. (25)
Year published	1992	1994	1995	1996
Therapy	Antidepressant	Topical capsaicin	Anticonvulsant	Antidepressant
Randomized, controlled trials reviewed, n	1	4	3	13
Outcome measure	Not specifically stated	Analgesic effectiveness (ascertained by physician)	>50% pain relief (ascertained by patient)	>50% pain relief (ascertained by patient)
Patients receiving active therapy who improved/all patients receiving active therapy, n/n	7/12[†]	105/144	56/58	180/260
Patients receiving placebo who improved/all patients receiving placebo, n/n	0/12[†]	81/165	29/68	73/205
Effect size	1.71			
Odds ratio (95% CI)		2.7 (1.7–4.9)	6.2 (3.0–10.6)	3.6 (2.5–5.2)
Number needed to treat (95% CI)		4.2 (2.9–7.5)[†]	2.5 (1.8–4.0)	2.9 (2.4–4.0)
Number needed to harm for minor adverse events (95% CI)			3.1 (2.3–4.8)	2.8 (2.0–4.7)
Number needed to harm for major adverse events (95% CI)			20 (10–446)	19 (11–74)

*Review of antidepressant agents in all chronic pain conditions.
[†]Calculated from information in the review but not included in the original review.

is is to assess the risk at baseline (the risk for a bad outcome without treatment) for a particular patient, but this assessment is even more important in prophylaxis because a very low risk for a bad outcome at baseline makes prophylaxis difficult to justify. We must sometimes make that judgment ourselves and subsequently adjust risks and balance benefits and potential harms on the basis of experience, although we can often use evidence from other sources. In assessing the risk for gastrointestinal bleeding from nonsteroidal anti-inflammatory drugs, for example, a large randomized study (19) tells us that elderly persons who have a history of peptic ulcer, gastrointestinal disease, or heart disease are at the highest risk. The decision of whether to use prophylactic gastric protection will be guided by this information. Figure 3.1 shows some of the issues that are involved in making choices in prophylaxis.

An example for prophylaxis can be seen by a woman presenting to your office with a dog bite. Because she has been receiving long-term, moderately high-dose systemic steroid therapy for inflammatory bowel disease, you strongly suspect that the patient is immunocompromised. You are therefore concerned that she may be at increased risk for infection from the bite wound. The question is whether to give the

patient prophylactic antibiotics to prevent such an infection. We know from a quantitative systematic review of randomized, controlled trials that has studied this question that evidence of benefit exists, with an overall NNT of 16 (Table 3.1).

How can this information be applied to your patient? Because she is immunocompromised, the patient's risk for developing an infection if she is not treated with antibiotics (sometimes referred to as the patient's expected event rate [3]) is considerably higher than that of the patients who were not immunocompromised in the systematic review. The patient's expected event rate might be estimated to be about five times greater than the 16% average rate of infection in the review (although the risk varied between 3% and 46% in individual studies). Assuming that the relative risk reduction is the same for high and low untreated risk, the estimated NNT that corresponds to the patient's estimated event rate is 16 ÷ 5, or 3. Thus, although antibiotic prophylaxis against subsequent infection in dog bites may not be worthwhile in all patients (NNT of 16 for patients who were not immunocompromised), it may be appropriate for this particular patient (NNT, 3). As an aside, if infection rates from dog bites in our area were much higher than the 16% in the review and approached the highest value

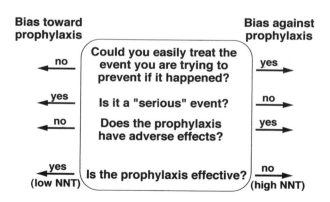

Figure 3.1 Issues involved in making choices in prophylaxis. NNT = number needed to treat.

that was found among the individual studies (50%), then we might be likely to give all patients prophylaxis with antibiotics.

Adverse and Other Events

The concepts that are captured by the NNT can also be used to express adverse events such as toxicity, side effects, or other harms. For minor adverse effects that are reported in randomized clinical trials, the NNH can be calculated in much the same way as the NNT. When the incidence of adverse events is low, it is likely that meaningful CIs will not be available (that is, the CIs may be infinite); therefore, only point estimates of harm will be available. Major harm may best be identified in randomized clinical trials through intervention-related withdrawal from the study; the NNH can be calculated from those numbers. Precise estimates of major harm often require a much wider literature search to find case reports or series, partly because these events are uncommon and partly because investigators may not report them in the full study, if they report them at all. The absence of information on adverse events in systematic reviews reduces the usefulness of such reviews (as in the case of topical capsaicin in Table 3.3).

Systematic reviews may also consider other consequences of treatment that may or may not be defined as adverse. A systematic review of the influence of epidural anesthesia during labor (27), for example, asked this question: If a woman is given epidural anesthesia, how much higher is her risk for having a cesarean section? In that review, a consistent increase in the rate of cesarean sections was noted in women who had epidural anesthesia. Sixteen percent of the women who had epidural anesthesia underwent cesarean sections compared with 6% of the women who did not have epidural anesthesia. The absolute risk increase was 10%, the relative risk increase was 161%, the NNT was 10 (CI, 8.4 to 13),

and the odds ratio (see below) was 2.6 (CI, 2.1 to 3.2). This means that for every 10 women in labor who are given epidural analgesia, 1 will have a cesarean section who otherwise would not have had the operation if she had received another form of analgesia. The NNT of 10 provides a figure that can be used by women and their caregivers in making choices about their labor.

Calculating Numbers Needed To Treat If They Are Not Provided

For statistical reasons, event rates in two groups are often compared in terms of odds ratios rather than relative risks (or absolute risk reductions). Thus, whereas the risk for an event (probability) is expressed relative to a total universe of fixed size (for example, when 22 events occur in a population of 100 persons, the risk for that event is 0.22), the odds of that same event in that same population are calculated as the number of events relative to the number of non-events (for example, 22 to 78, or 0.28). An odds ratio, then, is simply the odds of an event in a treatment group divided by the odds of the event in the comparison group. If a quantitative systematic review produces odds ratios but no NNTs, the NNT can be derived from the data in Figure 3.2.

The easiest way to use Figure 3.2 is first to choose the column nearest the published odds ratio and the row closest to the event rate expected and then to read the corresponding NNT. Note that the odds ratios in the left section of Figure 3.2 are less than 1.0, meaning that the outcome of interest in the active treatment group is less common than in the comparison group; this is the situation in prophylaxis (in which the outcome is onset, recurrence, or worsening of disease). In contrast, the odds ratios in the right section are greater than 1.0, meaning that the outcome of interest is more common in the treatment group; this is the

Odds Ratio

	Preventive Intervention									Treatment								
Control Event Rate	0.5	0.55	0.6	0.65	0.7	0.75	0.8	0.85	0.9	1.5	2	2.5	3	3.5	4	4.5	5	10
0.05	41	46	52	59	69	83	104	139	209	43	22	15	12	9	8	7	6	3
0.1	21	24	27	31	36	43	54	73	110	23	12	9	7	6	5	4	4	2
0.2	11	13	14	17	20	24	30	40	61	14	8	5	4	4	3	3	3	2
0.3	8	9	10	12	14	18	22	30	46	11	6	5	4	3	3	3	3	2
0.4	7	8	9	10	12	15	19	26	40	10	6	4	4	3	3	3	3	2
0.5	6	7	8	9	11	14	18	25	38	10	6	5	4	4	3	3	3	2
0.7	6	7	9	10	13	16	20	28	44	13	8	7	6	5	5	5	5	4
0.9	12	15	18	22	27	34	46	64	101	32	21	17	16	14	14	13	13	11

Figure 3.2 Calculation of the number needed to treat (NNT) from odds ratios. Table for estimating the NNT when the odds ratio (OR) and control event rate (CER) are known, published for preventive interventions in reference 28. The formula for determining the NNT for preventive interventions is {1 − [CER × (1 − OR)]}/[(1 − CER) × CER × (1 − OR)]. For treatment, the formula is [CER (OR − 1) + 1]/[CER (OR − 1) × (1 − CER)].

usual situation in studies of disease treatment (in which the outcome is cure, remission, or control of disease).

Figure 3.2 can also be used to determine how different values for event rate affect the NNT at a given odds ratio. Thus, if the rate of infection from dog bites in our area was 50%, then the NNT declines to 7 instead of 16 at an event rate of 16%. In such circumstances, as noted above, we might wish to use prophylactic antibiotics even for patients who are not immunocompromised.

As another example, the risk for cesarean section after epidural anesthesia, as noted above, has an odds ratio of 2.6; the event rate without epidural anesthesia is 6%. Using the odds ratios column of 2.5 and the event rate rows of 0.05 and 0.01 in Figure 3.2 yields an NNT somewhere between 9 and 15. This is close to the calculated figure of 10.

Odds ratios should be interpreted with caution when particular outcomes occur commonly, as in treatments for disease; odds ratios may then overestimate the effect of a treatment. Odds ratios are therefore likely to be replaced by relative risk reduction because relative risk reduction is more robust when event rates are high (3, 29). If relative risk reduction is provided in a review, NNT can be estimated from a useful nomogram (30).

Variation in Occurrence of Events

The incidence of events in a comparison group can and does vary, often widely, from study to study. For example, in trials of droperidol to prevent vomiting after surgery for correction of strabismus, the incidence of postoperative vomiting varied enormously (13) (Table 3.2). In some trials, almost no postoperative vomiting occurred; in others, the incidence was greater than 50% with the same operation and nearly identical anesthetics. Wide variation in event rates occurs with treatment and with prophylaxis. In six trials of natural surfactant for preterm infants, the event rate for bronchopulmonary dysplasia was 24% to 69% (31). Under other circumstances, the variation in event rate may be narrower. For example, the rate of ulcer healing without antibiotic treatment ranged from 0% to 17%

in 11 randomized, controlled trials that studied the therapeutic effect of eradicating *H. pylori* infection with antibiotics on ulcer healing (5).

The effectiveness of prophylaxis and treatment depends on the risk for the event without the active intervention. Thus, if patients do not vomit at baseline, then prophylaxis is not necessary; if most of them vomit, then prophylaxis may be particularly useful. If patients rarely recover from a disease without treatment, then treatment may be highly appropriate; if most patients recover on their own, then treatment may or may not be useful. The patient's expected event rate thus becomes important for the therapeutic or preventive decision, even when an intervention is proven to be effective.

Comments

A systematic review that is done properly can locate most of the useful information that has been published on a medical intervention. Such a compendium of information provides much more power than is often available from single trials because trials, particularly those that evaluate treatments, are often conducted with few patients in the experimental and comparison groups. During use of the results from systematic reviews, however, it is important to be able to shift from the numbers that are generally used to express the amount of benefit or harm from an intervention to a number that captures the effort that is necessary to achieve that benefit (or avoid that harm) in a given patient. Distilling the results of systematic reviews into, in effect, one number (the NNT or NNH) provides a measure of that effort and is therefore a clinically relevant approach. Physicians and patients can use this approach to rapidly estimate the amount of benefit and any accompanying harm for a given intervention. These calculations are simple to remember and use in personal or institu-

tional practice; they should help us to make the best possible clinical decisions with our patients.

Like all research results, however, NNTs are only one element of decision making and need to be integrated with patient preferences, caregiver experience and judgment, and local constraints and conditions. It is also worth noting that when clinicians and policymakers were presented with research results in different formats (NNT and absolute and relative risk reduction, among others), they made more conservative decisions when they received treatment effects expressed as NNTs than when they received them as relative risk reductions or absolute risk reductions (32-34).

Key Points To Remember

- Systematic reviews have the ability to produce the best evidence-based estimates of the true clinical effect of an intervention.
- As with individual clinical research studies, the various forms of numerical results from systematic reviews can easily be converted into a common currency, the number needed to treat.
- The number needed to treat is a clinically useful measure of the effort required to obtain a beneficial outcome with an intervention.
- The same concept can be applied to adverse outcomes, in which it becomes the number needed to harm.

Glossary

Relative risk: Risk for achieving an event (with treatment) or preventing an event (with prophylaxis) in the treatment group relative to that in the control group.

Relative risk reduction or increase: Increase in events with treatment compared with control (treatment) or reduction in events with treatment compared with control (prophylaxis); this number is often expressed as a percentage.

Absolute risk reduction: Difference in event rates for two groups, usually treatment and control.

Number needed to treat: Number of persons who must be treated for a given period to achieve an event (treatment) or to prevent an event (prophylaxis). The NNT is the reciprocal of the absolute risk reduction.

For more information, see References 1 to 3.

Acknowledgments: The authors thank David Sackett and Iain Chalmers for providing helpful comments, and Clifton Cleaveland, the clinical reviewer.

References

1. **Laupacis A, Sackett DL, Roberts RS.** An assessment of clinically useful measures of the consequences of treatment. N Engl J Med. 1988;318:1728-33.
2. **Cook RJ, Sackett DL.** The number needed to treat: a clinically useful measure of treatment effect. BMJ. 1995;310:452-4.
3. **Sackett D, Richardson WS, Rosenberg W, Haynes B.** Evidence Based Medicine. London: Churchill Livingstone; 1996.
4. **Vander Stichele RH, Dezeure EM, Bogaert MG.** Systematic review of clinical efficacy of topical treatments for head lice. BMJ. 1995;311:604-8.
5. **Moore RA.** *Helicobacter pylori* and peptic ulcer. A systematic review of effectiveness and an overview of the economic benefits of implementing what is known to be effective Oxford: Health Technology Evaluation Association; 1995. Available from http://www.jr2.ox.ac.uk/Bandolier/bandopubs/hpyl/hp0.html.
6. **Tfelt-Hansen P.** Sumatriptan for the treatment of migraine attacks: a review of controlled clinical studies. Cephalalgia. 1993;13:238-44.
7. **Haneke E, Tausch I, Bräutigam M, Weidinger G, Welzel D.** Short-duration treatment of fingernail dermatophytosis: a randomized, double-blind study with terbinafine and griseofulvin. J Am Acad Dermatol. 1995;32:72-7.
8. **Moore A, Collins S, Carroll D, McQuay H.** Paracetamol with and without codeine in acute pain: a quantitative systematic review. Pain. 1997; [In press].
9. **Laine L, Cook D.** Endoscopic ligation compared with sclerotherapy for treatment of esophageal variceal bleeding. A meta-analysis. Ann Intern Med. 1995;123:280-7.
10. **Rosenfeld RM, Vertrees JE, Carr J, Cipolle RJ, Uden DL, Giebink GS, et al.** Clinical efficacy of antimicrobial drugs for acute otitis media: meta-analysis of 5400 children from thirty-three randomized trials. J Pediatr. 1994;124:355-67.
11. **Lehert P, Comte S, Gamand S, Brown TM.** Naftidrofuryl in intermittent claudication: a retrospective analysis. J Cardiovasc Pharmacol. 1994; 23(Suppl 3):S48-52.
12. **Hazell P, O'Connell D, Heathcote D, Robertson J, Henry D.** Efficacy of tricyclic drugs in treating child and adolescent depression: a meta-analysis. BMJ. 1995;310:897-901.
13. **Tramer M, Moore A, McQuay H.** Prevention of vomiting after paediatric strabismus surgery: a systematic review using the numbers-needed-to-treat method. Br J Anaesth. 1995;75:556-61.
14. **Wells PS, Lensing AW, Hirsh J.** Graduated compression stockings in the prevention of postoperative venous thromboembolism. A meta-analysis. Arch Intern Med. 1994;154:67-72.
15. **Crowley PA.** Antenatal corticosteroid therapy: a meta-analysis of the randomized trials, 1972 to 1994. Am J Obstet Gynecol. 1995;173:322-35.
16. **Cummings P.** Antibiotics to prevent infection in patients with dog bite wounds: a meta-analysis of randomized trials. Ann Emerg Med. 1994;23:535-40.
17. **Mulrow CD, Cornell JA, Herrera CR, Kadri A, Farnett L, Aguilar C.** Hypertension in the elderly. Implications and generalizability of randomized trials. JAMA. 1994;272:1932-8.
18. Randomised trial of intravenous streptokinase, oral aspirin, both, or neither among 17,187 cases of suspected acute myocardial infarction: ISIS-2. ISIS-2 (Second International Study of Infarct Survival) Collaborative Group. Lancet. 1988;2: 349-60.
19. **Silverstein FE, Graham DY, Senior JR, Davies HW, Struthers BJ, Bittman RM, et al.** Misoprostol reduces serious gastrointestinal complications in patients with rheumatoid arthritis receiving nonsteroidal anti-inflammatory drugs. A randomized, double-blind, placebo-controlled trial. Ann Intern Med. 1995;123:241-9.
20. **Lancaster T, Silagy C, Gray S.** Primary care management of acute herpes zoster: systematic review of evidence from randomized controlled trials. Br J Gen Pract. 1995;45:39-45.
21. **Tfelt-Hansen P, Henry P, Mulder LJ, Scheldewaert RG, Schoenen J, Chazot G.** The effectiveness of combined oral lysine acetylsalicylate and metoclopramide compared with oral sumatriptan for migraine. Lancet. 1995;346:923-6.
22. **Onghena P, Van Houdenhove B.** Antidepressant-induced analgesia in chronic non-malignant pain: a meta-analysis of 39 placebo-controlled studies. Pain. 1992;49:205-19.
23. **Zhang WY, Li Wan Po A.** The effectiveness of topically applied capsaicin. A meta-analysis. Eur J Clin Pharmacol. 1994;46:517-22.
24. **McQuay H, Carroll D, Jadad AR, Wiffen P, Moore A.** Anticonvulsant drugs for management of pain: a systematic review. BMJ. 1995;311:1047-52.

25. **McQuay HJ, TramËr M, Nye BA, Carroll D, Wiffen PJ, Moore RA.** A systematic review of antidepressants in neuropathic pain. Pain. 1996;68:217-27.
26. **Gotzsche PC.** Sensitivity of effect variables in rheumatoid arthritis: a meta-analysis of 130 placebo controlled NSAID trials. J Clin Epidemiol. 1990;43:1313-8.
27. **Morton SC, Williams MS, Keeler EB, Gambone JC, Kahn KL.** Effect of epidural analgesia for labor on the cesarean delivery rate. Obstet Gynecol. 1994;83:1045-52.
28. **Sackett DL, Deeks JJ, Altman DG.** Down with odds ratios! Evidence-Based Medicine. 1996;1:164-6.
29. **Sinclair JC, Bracken MB.** Clinically useful measures of effect in binary analyses of randomized trials. J Clin Epidemiol. 1994;47:881-9.
30. **Chatellier G, Zapletal E, Lemaitre D, Menard J, Degoulet P.** The number needed to treat: a clinically useful nomogram in its proper context. BMJ. 1996;312:426-9.
31. **Soll JC, McQueen MC.** Respiratory distress syndrome. In: Sinclair JC, Bracken ME, eds. Effective Care of the Newborn Infant. New York: Oxford Univ Pr; 1992:333.
32. **Naylor CD, Chen E, Strauss B.** Measured enthusiasm: does the method of reporting trial results alter perceptions of therapeutic effectiveness? Ann Intern Med. 1992;117:916-21.
33. **Fahey T, Griffiths S, Peters TJ.** Evidence based purchasing: understanding results of clinical trials and systematic reviews. BMJ. 1995;311:1056-60.
34. **Bobbio M, Demichelis B, Giustetto G.** Completeness of reporting trial results: effect on physicians' willingness to prescribe. Lancet. 1994;343:1209-11.

Chapter 4

Using Systematic Reviews in Clinical Education

Robert G. Badgett, MD; Mary O'Keefe, MD; and Mark C. Henderson, MD

Traditional educational methods change clinical practice only with considerable effort and difficulty. In particular, the teaching of critical appraisal in the setting of journal clubs does not increase the amount of medical research read by trainees. Experiential learning theory, corroborated by the success of problem-based learning, encourages us to link learning to the numerous medical questions that physicians generate while providing patient care. Systematic reviews can link these questions with the results of research that would otherwise be difficult to locate, read, and appraise.

Systematic reviews are a uniquely powerful mechanism for teaching, and they offer teachers a new opportunity to model rational and effective use of information. Systematic reviews should be made available at clinical sites for use during "teachable moments." Resistance to the use of systematic reviews can be reduced by using existing journal clubs to teach about the strengths and limitations of these reviews. The point that systematic reviews are meant to assist, not replace, clinical decision making deserves emphasis in such teaching.

You are on rounds while attending on the wards when your team learns that a patient with septic shock is being admitted. The intern wants to begin therapy with corticosteroids, but the supervising resident is not sure whether that will help. While your team leaves to assess and stabilize the patient, you power up the computer in the conference room. You first execute a previously saved, structured MEDLINE search for *systematic reviews* and then combine the results of this search with articles containing the text words *septic shock*. You obtain several promising citations and, after reading the online abstracts, you conclude that steroids will not help and may even be harmful (1-3). Equipped with this up-to-date information, you quickly advise your team to delay using steroids until you can retrieve the relevant articles. After the patient is stabilized, you quickly read several of the articles and decide against using steroids.

Later that afternoon, you are supervising a busy clinic of internal medicine residents. A well-read senior resident asks about the efficacy of screening for ovarian cancer. While perusing the U.S. Preventive Service Task Force guidelines (4), you instruct the resident to look up the answer in the Canadian Guide to Clinical Preventive Health Care (5). Each of you finds a systematic review concluding that current technology is not effective in screening for ovarian cancer. The quick, comprehensive summaries of the literature impress the resident so much that she asks you to give a talk on cancer screening. You realize that this would be an excellent opportunity to teach trainees how systematic reviews can help them quickly locate high-quality answers to clinical problems. You plan to start the talk by outlining efficient methods with which to search for medical evidence.

Thinking back on these clinical teaching situations, you reflect that as you formulated your answers to the various queries, you suspected that many germane studies existed but you knew you would have insufficient time to review them individually. An organized and easily accessible synthesis of pertinent studies offered an excellent solution to this problem. In this chapter, we discuss how systematic reviews can enhance medical training by efficiently linking medical research with the many clinical questions that arise during patient care. We discuss how to facilitate the location of systematic reviews by trainees and how faculty can model the efficient location and use of these reviews. Finally, we discuss solutions to potential barriers, such as faculty reluctance to use systematic reviews and the difficulty in distinguishing high-quality systematic reviews from other types of reviews.

How Are Systematic Reviews Useful in Medical Training?

Traditional methods for keeping up with the burgeoning medical literature unfortunately do not increase the use of the literature by trainees (6-8). For many years, we have urged physicians in training (and in practice) to read original research. We have used journal clubs to teach critical appraisal and to model how we as clinician-educators keep up with research. However, the impact of journal clubs on resident behavior has been disappointing (6-8). Furthermore, neither trainees (9) nor faculty (10) want the faculty to attend journal clubs, and this reduces the opportunity to model efficient and effective use of the medical literature. Sadly, mandatory attendance and the provision of lunch are better than educational attributes at predicting which journal clubs will be well attended and will endure (9).

Many physicians in practice (11, 12) and in training (7) prefer to read traditional narrative review articles rather than original research studies. Previous authors in this series (13) and others (14-17) have discussed the scientific advantages that systematic reviews have over traditional reviews. We limit our discussion here to the characteristics of systematic reviews that are pertinent to medical education.

Systematic reviews can enhance training in several ways beyond providing trainees with reliable summaries of medical knowledge. First, a concise source of relevant evidence, such as that found in a systematic review, can encourage learning; in contrast, the time and effort involved in reading multiple original studies may discourage learning. Second, systematic reviews can help locate original studies when the trainee is not proficient in the electronic searching of the literature (18) or when the studies have not been published (19). Similarly, systematic reviews can serve as an interface between original research and trainees who may be inexperienced at critical appraisal. This can mitigate, in part, concerns about trainees reading secondary rather than primary research publications. Third, exposing trainees to systematic reviews may decrease the knowledge gap between trainees and their teachers, increasing the trainees' confidence and fostering active learning behavior. If trainees share systematic reviews with their teachers, mutual learning may occur because faculty knowledge is often less extensive outside of specific areas of expertise. Finally, the Residency Review Commission for internal medicine (20) strongly encourages residents to participate in scholarly activity during training. The Commission and many residency program directors (20) consider the preparation of "analytic" reviews to be scholarly activity.

Limitations of Systematic Reviews as Educational Resources

It is late 1995, and a patient presents with severe alcoholic hepatitis, encephalopathy, and no gastrointestinal bleeding. You advise your ward team to use steroids because a recent meta-analysis (21) and a subsequent well-executed trial (22) both conclude that steroids reduce mortality in such patients. The team uses steroids on the basis of your suggestion, but the patient dies 5 days later of septic shock. A few months later, your resident shows you the current issue of *ACP Journal Club* (23), which contains an abstract from a more recent meta-analysis concluding that steroids do not help patients with alcoholic hepatitis. You worry not only that the steroids may have contributed to the patient's death from sepsis (1) but may not even have been indicated for alcoholic hepatitis (23). This meta-analysis had been published before the patient died, and now you wonder whether you misinformed your ward team.

This scenario illustrates some of the limitations of systematic reviews. Trainees need to understand these limitations to use systematic reviews appropriately. Methodologic errors, and even bias, occur in systematic reviews just as they do in traditional reviews (24-26). Different systematic reviews on the same topic may produce conflicting conclusions (27, 28), as might be expected with any new and rapidly evolving scientific method. Residents must therefore learn to assess the quality of systematic reviews in order to understand why they may conflict with each other (27, 28) or with the results of individual randomized trials (29).

Ways To Incorporate Systematic Reviews into Medical Training

The most obvious way to incorporate systematic reviews into clinical training is at the bedside. Traditionally, much of medical education has consisted of the use of passive learning techniques, such as lectures and rounds scattered among patient encounters. However, experiential learning theory (30), which is corroborated by the success of problem-based learning (31), holds that learning should be more directly linked to clinical encounters. This grounding automatically creates a curriculum that is germane to clinical practice and thus increases learner motivation. Research has shown that physicians in training (32) and in practice (12) generate abundant questions while caring for patients. Unfortunately, many of these "teachable moments" are missed because attending physicians do not seek answers or refer to information resources that are convenient but less than reliable (12, 33, 34). Expeditious ways of seeking medical evidence, such as using systematic reviews, may increase the amount of learning done during clinical work and may improve clinical care at the same time.

Teachers can accomplish much by modeling the behavior we want our trainees to adopt, at the bedside or in the classroom (Table 4.1). We should model thoughtful searching for evidence rather than the "flash" retrieval of medical trivia from memory. A thoughtful approach teaches trainees both the value and the pleasure of searching for answers rather than maintaining a static knowledge base. Expediting the search for evidence by referring to systematic reviews strikes a balance between scientific rigor and the time pressures of clinical practice. We suggest the following examples of effective modeling.

At prepared conferences, teachers should cite systematic reviews whenever possible as sources of information. If none exist, a teacher may still stress their importance by noting this lack. In less structured situations, such as on ward rounds or in clinic, faculty should also model the use of systematic reviews. When questions arise that require less familiar information, the teacher can set about pursuing the evidence as described in the clinical scenarios at the beginning of this paper. If a current systematic review is not readily available in a textbook or article file, the teacher can try to locate one by using a previously saved literature search strategy, such as the computer-based strategy described by Hunt and McKibbon in chapter 2 (35). If the answer is not needed immediately, someone (including the teacher) can be assigned to bring a systematic review to the next session. We have found it efficient to place in our teaching computers a previously saved search strategy for locating systematic reviews. Trainees can download the strategy onto a floppy disk for use at home. Librarians can, of course, provide important help in searching for and in teaching persons how to search for systematic reviews. The librarians at the University of Rochester and at our institution have agreed to place previously saved

search strategies, including the strategy for locating systematic reviews, on a network server so that they are readily available to users on and off campus.

The following methods may facilitate the use of systematic reviews in your practice and teaching (Chapter 2 discusses some of these methods in more detail [35]). First, work to increase the availability of systematic reviews in all clinical settings. We suggest that teachers obtain and use the resources cited in Table 4.1. For example, many clinical sites already have files of frequently used articles. Systematic reviews should be included to the maximum possible extent in such files. Second, compilations of systematic reviews published as books or monographs, such as those published by the U.S. Preventive Services Task Force (4) (Table 4.1), are convenient if purchased but difficult to locate in journals. Another way to access systematic reviews is through the use of nonprint media. For example, the Internet provides access to the U.S. Preventive Services Task Force, the Agency for Health Care Policy and Research, and Canadian Guidelines (Table 4.1). Accessing the Internet quickly during clinical care is difficult to do without experience and an excellent dedicated computer system, but some reviews are available on disk. The Cochrane Library and the American College of Physicians position papers, which are accompanied by systematic reviews, can be purchased through the College. The College also sells Best Evidence, a CD-ROM that contains electronic versions of *ACP Journal Club* and *Evidence-Based Medicine*. Physicians can search this CD-ROM for meta-analyses, a common type of systematic review (Table 4.1).

As noted above, physicians can incorporate systematic reviews into training by encouraging residents to assist in performing one to fulfill the requirement for scholarly activity during training (36). This approach would enable trainees not only to gain clinical expertise in a given topic but to learn the methodology of systematic reviews. This will lead them to better understand the strengths and weaknesses of systematic reviews and how to apply these reviews in clinical problem solving.

Table 4.1   Incorporating Systematic Reviews into Medical Training by Modeling the Use of a Quick Strategy To Locate Them

1. Use quickly accessible books, monographs, and article files that contain systematic reviews

    Agency for Health Care Policy and Research, multiple practice guidelines (800-358-9295, ask for list)

    American College of Physicians, *Clinical Practice Guidelines* (800-523-1546)

    Consensus Conference on Antithrombotic Therapy, supplement published in *Chest* in October 1995

    Canadian Task Force on the Periodic Health Examination, *The Canadian Guide to Clinical Preventive Services* (819-956-4800)

    Rational Clinical Examination, a series of articles published in *Journal of the American Medical Association* since 1993

    U.S. Preventive Services Task Force, *Guide to Clinical Preventive Services* (800-638-0672)

2. If necessary, search the following databases, available on disk (all are available through the American College of Physicians at 800-523-1546):

    Best Evidence (CD-ROM version of *ACP Journal Club* and *Evidence-Based Medicine*)

    Cochrane Collaboration Library (includes the York Database of Reviews of Effectiveness)

3. If necessary, search the following databases, which are slower to use:

    MEDLINE*

    Internet resources†

    Agency for Health Care Policy and Research Clinical Practice Guidelines (http://text.nlm.nih.gov)

    Canadian Task Force on the Periodic Health Examination, Clinical Preventive Health Care (http://www.cma.ca/cpgs/by_dev.htm HCAN)

    U.S. Preventive Services Task Force Guide to Clinical Preventive Services (http://text.nlm.nih.gov)

*Commercial services for MEDLINE searching include Ovid (http://www.ovid.com) and Silver Platter (http://www.silverplatter.com). Combine your clinical topic with a previously saved, structured literature search for systematic reviews. A suggested strategy is detailed in Chapter 2 (35).
†The print versions of these guidelines can be assessed more quickly than the Internet versions.

Barriers and Possible Solutions to the Use of Systematic Reviews in Medical Education

Lack of faculty support is a major potential barrier to the use of systematic reviews in training. Nongeneralists tend to value these reviews less than generalists do (12). Furthermore, some teachers may feel threatened by systematic reviews, some of which may challenge their own opinions (37). In addition, faculty may not be convinced of the value of systematic reviews. The following approaches may reduce faculty (and trainee) reluctance to use systematic reviews.

First, it is critical to emphasize that systematic reviews are not meant to replace clinician decision making. Rather, clinicians should be encouraged to become authorities on the clinical interpretation and application of systematic reviews. Second, faculty must be convinced of the value of these reviews. Unfortunately, no studies have examined the impact of systematic reviews on medical education. One study (38) found that practicing physicians were not particularly interested in using systematic reviews. However, this study is now several years old, and the exponential increase in the publication rate of systematic reviews means that they are now available for many clinical questions. When interpreting the results of this study, one should also realize that educating practicing physicians is generally not an effective way to change clinical practice (39). This may support the use of systematic reviews during training because trainees may be more open to new ways of learning. Faculty may be less reluctant to use systematic reviews if they realize that producers of evidence-based clinical guidelines (4, 40), "opinion leader" physicians (leaders in hospital staffs, medical communities, and professional societies and members of certification and editorial boards) (12), policymakers for health care plans (41), and even the insurance industry

(42) seek evidence from systematic reviews. We have observed that clinicians best learn the value of systematic reviews when they can readily locate one during a "teachable moment."

Faculty use of systematic reviews may be increased through use of the following strategies. First, subspecialty teachers can be recruited into locating pertinent systematic reviews for inclusion in teaching files (many of these reviews are published only in subspecialty journals). A jointly prepared bibliography that emphasizes systematic reviews can then be provided to trainees before subspecialty rotations are started. Second, trainees can serve as "vectors," spreading interest in and knowledge about the power and utility of systematic reviews. We can encourage trainees to solicit systematic reviews from all faculty, not just those who volunteer. Third, if a training program encourages residents to do systematic reviews to fulfill a requirement for scholarly work, the residents should solicit help from a wide variety of clinical faculty whose experience makes them content experts.

A second barrier is that trainees themselves do not understand the nature of systematic reviews. At our institution, we have modified our journal clubs so that they teach the strengths and limitations of systematic reviews. In addition, we teach brief guidelines on assessing the quality of systematic reviews (43), on distinguishing systematic from traditional reviews, and on efficiently searching MEDLINE for systematic reviews.

Authors of systematic reviews have an important role to play in facilitating the use of their work by trainees. Some systematic reviews are as tedious to read as original research articles. Authors should make their reviews easier to read and should use structured abstracts. Authors of systematic reviews, editors of medical journals, and custodians of such bibliographic databases

as MEDLINE must continue working to improve the identification of systematic reviews and their distinction from traditional reviews. For example, MEDLINE cannot recognize some excellent systematic reviews (40) because they do not have abstracts (44), Medical Subject Headings, or words in the titles that distinguish them from traditional reviews.

Several barriers may hinder trainees who are interested in performing systematic reviews. Possible solutions are discussed in detail elsewhere (45). Most important, residents need such resources as protected time, mentors, and methodologic instruction. Each training program should provide administrative time for a faculty member who is a designated coordinator of resident scholarly activity. This person can help trainees select feasible research questions and locate appropriate faculty mentors. Performing a systematic review correctly can be a demanding, complex, and frustrating exercise, and residents should not be expected to work alone on such a project. Thus, the coordinator should ensure that trainees receive both content-related and methodologic guidance. If the coordinator has expertise in performing systematic reviews, he or she can assist mentors who do not have experience. Alternatively, a subset of mentors could be trained by local experts or by programs such as the Cochrane Training workshop (46). Finally, the coordinator should encourage clinician educators to be mentors and should acknowledge the help of mentors to department chairpersons.

Conclusions

Systematic reviews are becoming—and should become—integral to the dissemination of medical knowledge to physicians in training and in practice. Systematic reviews organize the medical literature and, hence, provide an interface between the physician and original research. Teaching and modeling the use of systematic reviews will therefore improve physician training and true lifelong professional development. We believe that the acquisition of such skills will ultimately result in better patient care.

Key Points To Remember

- Traditional methods for keeping up with the literature, such as journal clubs and courses in critical appraisal, do not increase the amount of medical literature read by trainees.
- Systematic reviews may compensate for physicians' deficiencies in locating and appraising original research.
- Systematic reviews should be readily available at clinical sites for use during "teachable moments".
- Faculty members should model the use of systematic reviews in clinical decision making.
- Reluctance to use systematic reviews may be reduced by teaching the strengths and weaknesses of these reviews and by emphasizing that they are not meant to replace clinical decision making.

Appendix

To identify references used in this chapter 1) MEDLINE textword searches were done for each of the following: journal club, critical appraisal, grand rounds, dissemination, problem based learning; and 2) MEDLINE Medical Subject Heading searches were done separately for each of the following: databases, bibliographic and databases, electronic. In addition, a strategy similar to that described in reference 35 was combined with "septic shock.tw." or "diethylstilb$.tw." The 12/95 CD-ROM version of *ACP Journal Club* was searched for "meta-analyses." Additional sources included the following document: National Library of Medicine. Current bibliographies

in medicine: meta-analysis. Washington, DC: US Gov Pr Office; 1993.

Acknowledgment: The authors thank the clinical reviewer, Paul F. Speckart, MD.

References

1. **Cronin L, Cook DJ, Carlet J, Heyland DK, King D, Lansang MA, et al.** Corticosteroid treatment for sepsis: a critical appraisal and meta-analysis of the literature. Crit Care Med. 1995;23:1313-5.
2. **Lefering R, Neugebauer EA.** Steroid controversy in sepsis and septic shock: a meta-analysis. Crit Care Med. 1995;23:1294-303.
3. **Frey FJ, Speck RF.** [Glucocorticoids and infection.] Schweiz Med Wochenschr 1992;122:137-46.
4. Screening for ovarian cancer. In: U.S. Preventive Services Task Force. Guide to Clinical Preventive Services: Report of the U.S. Preventive Services Task Force. 2d ed. Baltimore: Williams & Wilkins; 1996:159-66.
5. Screening for ovarian cancer. In: Canadian Task Force on the Periodic Health Examination. The Canadian Guide to Clinical Preventive Health Care. Ottawa: Canada Communication Group; 1994:870-82.
6. **Audet N, Gagnon R, Ladouceur R, Marcil M.** L'enseignement de l'analyse critique des publications scientifiques mÈdicales est-il efficace? Révision des études et de leur qualité méthodologique. [How effective is the teaching of critical analysis of scientific publications? Review of studies and their methodological quality.] Can Med Assoc J. 1993;148:945-52.
7. **Landry FJ, Pangaro L, Kroenke K, Lucey C, Herbers J.** A controlled trial of a seminar to improve medical student attitudes toward, knowledge about, and use of the medical literature. J Gen Intern Med. 1994;9:436-9.
8. **Linzer M, Brown JT, Frazier LM, DeLong ER, Siegel WC.** Impact of a medical journal club on house-staff reading habits, knowledge, and critical appraisal skills. A randomized control trial. JAMA. 1988;260:2537-41.
9. **Sidorov J.** How are internal medicine residency journal clubs organized, and what makes them successful? Arch Intern Med. 1995;155:1193-7.
10. **Moberg-Wolff EA, Kosasih JB.** Journal clubs. Prevalence, format, and efficacy in PM&R. Am J Phys Med Rehabil. 1995;74:224-9.
11. **Curley SP, Connelly DP, Rich EC.** Physicians' use of medical knowledge resources: preliminary theoretical framework and findings. Med Decis Making. 1990;10:231-41.
12. **Williamson JW, German PS, Weiss R, Skinner EA, Bowes F 3d.** Health science information management and continuing education of physicians. A survey of U.S. primary care practitioners and their opinion leaders. Ann Intern Med. 1989;110:151-60.

13. **Cook DJ, Mulrow CD, Haynes RB.** Systematic reviews: synthesis of best evidence for clinical decisions. Ann Intern Med. 1997;126:376-80.

14. **Antman EM, Lau J, Kupelnick B, Mosteller F, Chalmers TC.** A comparison of results of meta-analyses of randomized control trials and recommendations of clinical experts. Treatments for myocardial infarction. JAMA. 1992;268:240-8.

15. **Neihouse PF, Priske SC.** Quotation accuracy in review articles. DICP. 1989;23:594-6.

16. **Oxman AD, Guyatt GH.** The science of reviewing research. Ann N Y Acad Sci. 1993;703:125-34.

17. **Mulrow CD.** The medical review article: state of the science. Ann Intern Med. 1987;106:485-8.

18. **Haynes RB, McKibbon KA, Walker CJ, Ryan N, Fitzgerald D, Ramsden MF.** Online access to MEDLINE in clinical settings. A study of use and usefulness. Ann Intern Med. 1990;112:78-84.

19. **Cook DJ, Guyatt GH, Ryan G, Clifton J, Buckingham L, Willan A, et al.** Should unpublished data be included in meta-analyses? Current convictions and controversies. JAMA. 1993;269:2749-53.

20. **Alguire PC, Anderson WA, Albrecht RR, Poland GA.** Resident research in internal medicine training programs. Ann Intern Med. 1996;124:321-8.

21. **Imperiale TF, McCullough AJ.** Do corticosteroids reduce mortality from alcoholic hepatitis? A meta-analysis of the randomized trials. Ann Intern Med. 1990;113:299-307.

22. **Ramond MJ, Poynard T, Rueff B, Mathurin P, Theodore C, Chaput J, et al.** A randomized trial of prednisolone in patients with severe alcoholic hepatitis. N Engl J Med. 1992;326:507-12.

23. Glucocorticosteroids are probably ineffective in alcoholic hepatitis [Abstract]. ACP J Club. 1996;124:13.

24. **Sacks HS, Berrier J, Reitman D, Ancona-Berk VA, Chalmers TC.** Meta-analyses of randomized controlled trials. N Engl J Med. 1987;316:450-5.

25. **Macarthur C, Foran PJ, Bailar JC 3d.** Qualitative assessment of studies included in a meta-analysis: DES and the risk of pregnancy loss. J Clin Epidemiol. 1995;48:739-47.

26. **Bailar JC 3d.** The practice of meta-analysis. J Clin Epidemiol. 1995;48:149-57.

27. **Messer J, Reitman D, Sacks HS, Smith H Jr, Chalmers TC.** Association of adrenocorticosteroid therapy and peptic-ulcer disease. N Engl J Med. 1983;309:21-4.

28. **King PD.** Glucocorticosteroids are probably ineffective in alcoholic hepatitis [Commentary]. ACP Journal Club. 1996;124:13.

29. **Collins R, Peto R, Steight P.** ISIS-4 [Letter]. Lancet. 1995;345:1374-5.

30. The process of experiential learning. In: Kolb DA. Experiential Learning: Experience as the Source of Learning and Development. Englewood Cliffs, NJ: Prentice-Hall; 1984:20-38.

31. **Vernon DT, Blake RL.** Response to "Problem-based learning: have expectations been met?" [Letter] Acad Med. 1995;69:472-3.

32. **Osheroff JA, Forsythe DE, Buchanan BG, Bankowitz RA, Blumenfeld BH, Miller RA.** Physicians' information needs: analysis of questions posed during clinical teaching. Ann Intern Med. 1991;114:576-81.

33. **Covell DG, Uman GC, Manning PR.** Information needs in office practice: are they being met? Ann Intern Med. 1985;103:596-9.

34. **Avorn J, Chen M, Hartley R.** Scientific versus commercial sources of influence on the prescribing behavior of physicians. Am J Med. 1982;73:4-8.

35. **Hunt DL, McKibbon KA.** Locating and appraising systematic reviews. Ann Intern Med. 1997;126:532-538.

36. **Davidoff F.** Who Has Seen a Blood Sugar? Reflections on Medical Education. Philadelphia: American Coll Physicians; 1996:44.

37. **Rosenberg W, Donald A.** Evidence based medicine: an approach to clinical problem-solving. BMJ. 1995;310:1122-6.

38. **Paterson-Brown S, Fisk NM, Wyatt JC.** Uptake of meta-analytical overviews of effective care in English obstetric units. Br J Obstet Gynaecol. 1995;102:297-301.

39. **Davis DA, Thomson MA, Oxman AD, Haynes RB.** Changing physician performance. A systematic review of the effect of continuing medical education strategies. JAMA. 1995;274:700-5.

40. **Dalen JE, Hirsh J.** Introduction. In: 4th American College of Chest Physicians Consensus Conference on Antithrombotic Therapy. Tucson, Arizona, April 1995. Proceedings. Chest. 1995;108:225S-6S.

41. **Steiner CA, Powe NR, Anderson GF, Das A.** The review process used by US health care plans to evaluate new medical technology for coverage. J Gen Intern Med. 1996;11:294-302.

42. **Anderson C.** Congress looks for methods to assess clinical research. Nature. 1992;357:5.

43. **Oxman AD, Cook DJ, Guyatt GH.** Users' guides to the medical literature. VI: How to use an overview. Evidence-Based Medicine Working Group. JAMA. 1994;272:1367-71.

44. **Haynes RB, Mulrow CD, Huth EJ, Altman DG, Gardner MJ.** More informative abstracts revisited. Ann Intern Med. 1990;113:69-76.

45. **Schultz HJ.** Research during internal medicine residency training: meeting the challenge of the Residency Review Committee [Editorial]. Ann Intern Med. 1996;124:340-2.

46. **Mulrow CD, Oxman AD, eds.** Cochrane Collaboration Handbook [updated 21 October 1996]. In: The Cochrane Library [database on disk and CD-ROM]. The Cochrane Collaboration, Issue 3. London: BMJ; 1996. Updated quarterly.

Chapter 5

How Consumers and Policymakers Can Use Systematic Reviews for Decision Making

Lisa A. Bero, PhD; and Alejandro R. Jadad, MD, DPhil

Systematic reviews can be very useful decision-making tools because they objectively summarize large amounts of information, identify gaps in medical research, and identify beneficial or harmful interventions. Consumers can use systematic reviews to help them make health care decisions. Policymakers can use systematic reviews to help them make decisions about what types of health care to provide. Despite the potential value of systematic reviews, little evidence of their direct impact on the decisions made by consumers and policymakers is available. We discuss strategies for optimizing the use of systematic reviews by increasing the awareness and identification of reviews, learning to critically evaluate the findings of reviews, and overcoming barriers to the incorporation of reviews into the decision-making process. In addition, the participation of consumers and policymakers in the design, conduct, and reporting of systematic reviews can help to produce reviews that are relevant and understandable to target audiences. Because decisions that involve health care policies and issues are complex processes in which information (such as that provided by systematic reviews) plays only a part, strategies for increasing the use of systematic reviews should be evaluated for their usefulness in the decision-making process.

A healthy pregnant woman is deciding whether she should have the ultrasonography recommended by her physician. Members of a city council are deciding whether to prohibit tobacco smoking in local restaurants and bars. Decisions such as these are made daily by health care consumers who must determine whether to have a diagnostic procedure or select one of several treatment alternatives, and by policymakers who must choose the types of health care to provide. In this chapter, we discuss how systematic reviews can help during the decision-making process. In our discussion, consumers include both patients and healthy persons, their family members, and their advocates. Policymakers include decision makers at the national, regional, local, and institutional levels. For example, administrators, local health authorities, purchasers of health care, and regulatory bodies are considered policymakers.

Our discussion concentrates on the factors that influence decisions common to both consumers and policymakers. However, one fundamental difference between the decision-making process of policymakers and that of patients and healthy persons is the tendency of policymakers to consider the perspective of the general population, whereas patients or healthy persons are obviously more likely to consider their own perspective. When making decisions, policymakers consider the burden of suffering, that is, the morbidity and mortality associated with a condition if a person does not receive treatment and the prevalence of a condition in the general population (1). If the burden of suffering is high, then policymakers may recommend action. Consumers, in contrast, are understandably more likely to consider personal suffering and benefits when making a decision. What may be best for the group may not necessarily be best for the individual (2).

Current Use of Systematic Reviews by Consumers and Policymakers

Our search for evaluations of the use of systematic reviews identified little published evidence to support the opinion that systematic reviews currently influence the medical or health care decisions made by the general public and by policymakers. We found only one study (3) in which systematic reviews influenced hypothetical decisions about reimbursement for mammography screening and cardiac rehabilitation and one case report (4) in which one of the authors conducted a systematic review that persuaded a physician to change his recommendations. The lack of research on the

impact that systematic reviews have on decision making may be the result of a lack of interest by the research community or the complexity of studying decision-making processes.

In our search, we attempted to identify studies that assessed the direct impact of systematic reviews on decisions made by policymakers and consumers. Although we only found two evaluations, the literature does offer numerous examples of how systematic reviews have been used to gather information for policymaking. For example, Light and Pillemer (5) describe how systematic reviews have been commissioned by policymakers to answer their questions. Guidelines on clinical practice (such as those from the Agency for Health Care Policy and Research and from the American College of Physicians) are often based on systematic reviews. In addition, technology assessments (such as those conducted by the U.S. Office of Technology Assessment) often include a systematic review of the literature on clinical efficacy as part of the assessment. We have learned that systematic reviews are more frequently cited than original research articles in coverage by the news media of research on the effects of environmental tobacco smoke; this fact suggests that systematic reviews might be indirectly influencing policy decisions as a result of such coverage (6). The use of systematic reviews in policy development reinforces the need to rigorously evaluate their direct impact on policy decisions.

Several factors may explain the reason that minimal data are available on the impact of systematic reviews on decisions made by policymakers and consumers. Decision makers consider the source, format, perceived relevance, and other aspects of information when making decisions (Table 5.1). The tendency of decision makers to use anecdotal aspects of the most recent evidence or personal experience rather than evaluate evidence broadly and systematically undermines the use of systematic reviews (7). In addition, the role of information depends on its interaction with other components of the decision-making process (including the values, preferences, and beliefs of the decision maker) and the context in which the decision is being made (Table 5.1) (8). Furthermore, although the methods for conducting systematic reviews have been available to the medical community for years, these reviews have only recently been applied to clinical care (12-14). For example, a landmark article summarizing the state of the science of systematic reviewing was published in the medical literature in 1987 (15). In addition, the Cochrane Collaboration, an international organization whose goal is to design, conduct, and disseminate systematic reviews in medicine, was founded in 1992 (16).

The role of information as only one aspect of the complex decision-making process is illustrated by our hypothetical examples. The healthy pregnant woman who is deciding whether to have ultrasonography should be interested to learn that four systematic reviews that assessed routine ultrasonography in early pregnancy have found the procedure to be safe and effective for detecting fetal malformations (17-20). However, she will probably weigh this information against her perceived risk for having a baby with a malformation, the amount of time she must take from work, the inconvenience associated with having ultrasonography (for example, out-of-pocket expenses), and the experience of her sister or next-door neighbor (21). In contrast, the members of a city council, while making their decision on whether to restrict tobacco smoking, can be informed by three meta-analyses of the effects of passive smoke on heart disease (22-24). However, council members are also likely to consider the opinions of their constituents and the pressures exerted by lobbyists for the tobacco industry and advocacy groups.

Table 5.1   Examples of Factors That Influence Decisions of Consumers and Policymakers*

Information

Source (for example, mass media, friends, support groups, professional organizations)

Clarity of contents

Formatting and framing (how information is presented)

Perceived validity

Perceived relevance

Strength of the message (vividness)

Personal values, preferences, and beliefs

Role of the decision maker (consumer or policy maker)

Socioeconomic background

Previous education or experience

Political affiliations

Willingness to adopt innovations

Willingness to accept uncertainty

Willingness to participate in decisions

Ethical aspects of the decision

Prior hypotheses

Context

Role of the decision maker (consumer or policy maker)

Culture

Lobbying by special-interest organizations

Timing

Administrative, financial, or political constraints

* Information obtained from References 7 through 11.

The Rationale for Using Systematic Reviews

Although information in any format plays only a limited (but potentially significant) role in the decision-making process, we have reason to believe that systematic reviews can have a particularly important influence on the decisions made by both consumers and policymakers. A properly conducted systematic review can provide an objective summary of large amounts of data. For consumers and policymakers who are interested in the bottom line of evidence, systematic reviews can help cohere conflicting results of research. Systematic reviews can form the basis for other integrative articles produced by policymakers, such as risk assessments, practice guidelines, economic analyses, and decision analyses (25). Systematic reviews can aid the process of consensus development by curtailing the criticism that consensus development tends to occur in the absence of an objective framework for collecting and reviewing evidence (1). Systematic reviews also typically identify gaps in knowledge, thereby helping consumers and policymakers decide not to proceed in the absence of evidence or encouraging them to address the gaps in medical research. Savulescu and colleagues (26) have recommended that medical ethics committees require researchers to conduct systematic reviews of existing relevant research to ensure the need for a new study.

As is true for the results of any research, however, inappropriate use of systematic reviews can result in more harm than good. Some of the risks of systematic reviews can be illustrated with our hypothetical example of the healthy pregnant woman. In the United Kingdom, leaflets that are targeted to pregnant women and health care professionals offer informed choice by reviewing the value of routine ultrasonography. The leaflets summarize systematic reviews of the best available evidence on the efficacy and safety of routine ultrasonography in pregnant women. In a case study on the reactions of women and health care professionals to the leaflets (27), women reacted with shock at the contents of the leaflets but were glad to be presented with the advantages and disadvantages of routine scanning and often requested additional information. Midwives believed that the leaflets would help women seek better health care, whereas ultrasonographers were concerned that the leaflets would provoke anxiety among women and lessen the use of routine ultrasonography

(27). The conflicting reactions of the midwives and ultrasonographers could lead to confrontation and lack of trust.

Additional harm could result from misrepresentation of the conclusions of systematic reviews to promote the self-interests of organizations or to support political positions. For example, a systematic review (24) of the cardiac effects of environmental tobacco smoke was presented without referring to other literature on the effects of passive smoking and was misconstrued as failing to conclude that environmental tobacco smoke is harmful (28). Misinterpretation of systematic reviews in the lay literature can affect the decisions made by government officials, including our hypothetical example of a city council regulating tobacco smoking.

Although the potential benefits of systematic reviews seem to outweigh the harms, sustained efforts are needed to increase our understanding of each stage involved in the use of systematic reviews as a decision-making tool (Table 5.2). In the following sections, we describe strategies for optimizing the use of systematic reviews by using a model analogous to that proposed for the study of the diffusion of innovations (9).

Optimizing the Use of Systematic Reviews

Increasing Access to Systematic Reviews: Awareness and Identification of Reviews

For systematic reviews to influence decisions, health care consumers and policymakers must first be aware of the existence, characteristics, and potential value of the reviews. Policymakers are usually knowledgeable about research that supports their policy positions (7). With increasing access to the Internet, consumers are also being exposed to information that

Table 5.2   Stages in the Use of Systematic
            Reviews by Consumers and
            Policymakers

Awareness of the existence of systematic reviews

Perception of the advantages and disadvantages of
    using them

Identification of individual reviews

Critical evaluation

Incorporation into decisions

Participating in the design, evaluation, and
    dissemination of findings

was previously inaccessible (29). It is unknown, however, how much consumers and policymakers know about systematic reviews, including where to find them.

Systematic reviews are often published in medical journals that can be identified through searches of bibliographic databases. Accessibility to systematic reviews could be improved if the reviews were available in the offices of policymakers, through public libraries, or by home computers. In addition, physicians could play a role in facilitating shared decision making by linking consumers to information in systematic reviews. One example of a nationwide effort to increase availability of reviews is practiced in the United Kingdom, where all hospitals, ambulance services, and community health care centers subscribe to the Cochrane Library, an electronic database of reviews published by the Cochrane Collaboration (30). Thus, health care policymakers in the United Kingdom have access to systematic reviews. The distribution of reasonably priced collections of systematic reviews by public and professional organizations could also increase awareness of reviews.

Networks of interested persons can improve access to systematic reviews. The Cochrane Consumer Network is an international network that facilitates dissemination of information from systematic reviews to consumers, their families, and their advocates by sharing information

among network members and notifying the news media of interesting developments (31). (For information on the Cochrane Consumer Network, contact Hilda Bastian, Coordinator, Consumer Network, The Australasian Cochrane Centre, Flinders Medical Centre, Bedford Park SA 5042, Australia. Telephone: 61 8 204 5399; fax: 61 8 276 3305 [e-mail: hilda.bastian@flinders.edu.au].) A network of clinical policymakers from key organizations has been proposed as a way to increase awareness of systematic reviews of pregnancy and childbirth among health care professionals (32).

Critical Evaluation of Systematic Reviews

All research may be perceived as being driven by the biases and vested interests of the researchers and funders (33). Systematic reviews, like other forms of research, vary in methodologic quality; biased reviews could lead to potentially damaging conclusions (34, 35). Therefore, health care consumers and policymakers should consider limiting their sources of information to the most rigorously conducted systematic reviews. Simple tools for critically appraising reviews and databases might include distinguishing systematic reviews from narrative reviews (36). Complete disclosure of funding sources and realization that authors may have conflicts of interest could also help consumers and policymakers select balanced systematic reviews (37). For example, in the hypothetical example of a city council making decisions about enacting restrictions on tobacco smoking, council members should know that some review articles on the health effects of passive smoking were sponsored by the tobacco industry. These articles found a lack of adverse health effects (even after controlling for quality or peer review) in contrast to the findings of review articles that were not sponsored by the tobacco industry (38).

Using Systematic Reviews for Decision Making

Even if health care consumers and policymakers are given understandable, timely, relevant, objective information, numerous other factors (such as those listed in Table 5.1) influence the incorporation of systematic reviews into the decision-making process. Barriers to the use of evidence when making decisions have been discussed extensively by other authors and are beyond the scope of this chapter (21, 39, 40). In brief, the use of systematic reviews can be increased relative to the use of personal value and contextual factors in making policy decisions by identifying the barriers that are specific to each target audience and designing focused strategies to overcome the barriers (10).

Participation in the Design and Reporting of Systematic Reviews

One major barrier to the use of systematic reviews by policymakers and consumers is that the information must be perceived as relevant to the decision at hand (21). Health care consumers and policymakers may regard academic research as irrelevant because it is not timely, asks the wrong questions, or is simply not interesting (41). Furthermore, because the research community controls the funding of a study, the manner in which the study is conducted, and the publication and dissemination of findings, consumers and policymakers have little opportunity to provide input.

The questions of researchers tend to differ from those of consumers and policymakers. To develop a focused research question, researchers may oversimplify the problem (42). In contrast, consumers and policymakers prefer to focus on more complex questions that address problems in the context of their local circumstances. In addition, researchers may concentrate on measurable, intermediate outcomes that are irrelevant to policymakers and consumers.

For example, outcomes that are relevant to persons who have heart failure might include mortality and health-related quality of life, but such outcomes as echocardiographic measurements or exercise-tolerance testing may not be of concern (43). Research often does not provide data on the relative costs of treatments or on direct comparisons of treatments. Some of the deficiencies of research could be addressed by involving health care consumers and policymakers in the design of primary studies (44, 45). For example, patients with cancer, their family members, and clinicians have worked together to identify, evaluate, and draw conclusions from relevant research, including systematic reviews, for developing a guide to the treatment of pain associated with cancer (46).

Systematic reviews with narrow research questions can assist policymakers and consumers if sufficient information has been provided to allow the decision maker to interpret the results. Systematic reviews that provide detailed information on the inclusion and exclusion criteria for original studies and an assessment of the characteristics of these studies can help consumers and policymakers determine whether the findings are helpful. For instance, in our example of a healthy pregnant woman who needs to decide whether to have ultrasonography, the women would be interested only in considering the results of systematic reviews that evaluated studies on the effects of ultrasonography in healthy women who had low-risk pregnancies.

Participatory approaches to research could produce systematic reviews that answer questions of greater relevance to consumers and policymakers than the questions now being addressed. The focus of participatory research is knowledge for action in contrast to knowledge for understanding (47). Participatory research uses a bottoms-up approach to planning that considers local priorities, processes, and perspectives. For example, the National Health Service in the United Kingdom has tried to incorporate policy and consumer input into research planning (48). Since 1991, the Service has conducted widespread consultations that have encouraged its own staff, statutory agencies, clinical management, professional bodies, consumer groups, academic centers, and research organizations to identify the needs for research, including systematic reviews.

Consumer and policymaker participation cannot, of course, correct the inadequacies that exist in the original research studies included in a systematic review. However, input from consumers and policymakers could ensure that the systematic review contains relevant information. In addition to commissioning topics for reviews (as encouraged by the National Health Service in the United Kingdom), consumers and policymakers could be educated to evaluate reviews critically and could use this capability to experiment with methods of interpreting and presenting the findings of systematic reviews. The Cochrane Collaboration provides unmatched opportunities for health care consumers to become involved in the design, interpretation, and use of the results of systematic reviews. Members of the Cochrane Consumer Network sit on the steering group of the Collaboration and, in increasing number, are joining the groups that are responsible for producing the reviews. Members of the Network are writing summaries of reviews that are targeted to a lay audience and are developing methods of disseminating the reviews to consumers. This involvement of consumers in such organizations as the Cochrane Collaboration could lead not only to more relevant research but also, in principle, to more efficient use of health care resources (31, 49).

Other factors that can influence decision making include how risk is reported (3) and the overall presentation of research results. The length of a report, the complexity of the language, the measurements used to express the outcomes, and the ease with which the bottom line is identified also can influence decision making. Executive summaries of systematic reviews that are developed specifically for (and, ideally, with) consumers and policymakers and that clearly and concisely state the results of these reviews could be useful in conveying their specialized information. The manner in which the summary is written should be intellectually accessible, relevant, and appealing. An example is the leaflets (developed in the United Kingdom) that summarized the result of systematic reviews of routine ultrasonography for health care consumers and professionals (27). Another potentially useful strategy would be electronic publication of jargon-free versions of systematic reviews with hypertext links that allow readers who have various academic backgrounds to access information at different levels of complexity.

Conclusion

Systematic reviews can be very useful decision-making tools by objectively summarizing large amounts of information, identifying gaps in medical research, and identifying beneficial or harmful interventions. To date, little published research has evaluated the direct impact of systematic reviews on the decisions made by health care consumers and policymakers. This scarcity of research could be explained, at least partially, by limited availability of reviews; lack of interest by researchers; lack of evidence that the information would be beneficial; and absence of strategies that increase the awareness of consumers and policymakers and improve the identification, appraisal, and application of systematic reviews. Ideally, when decision makers incorporate results of systematic reviews in their decisions, they would collaborate with researchers to assess the impact of this information on outcomes (9).

Making decisions on health care policies and issues is a complex process in which obtaining information plays only one part of the whole. Even if all existing barriers to the use of systematic reviews were overcome, these reviews would be an important, but not an obligatory or sufficient, component of decisions on health care (50, 51). Further efforts are required to improve our understanding of how various sources of information interact and how information is processed in different contexts by individuals with different values. In the meantime, efforts should continue to ensure that systematic reviews contain sufficient information on the reviews' methods and sponsorship and that they are presented in an accessible and appealing fashion that enables users to judge their validity and relevance.

Many of the current barriers to the use of systematic reviews by consumers and policymakers also affect clinicians and researchers. Time and effort would be wasted if each of these groups independently developed and evaluated strategies to overcome the common barriers. Finding the answers to the questions that are relevant to policymakers and consumers requires effective collaboration among all decision makers.

Key Points To Remember

- Systematic reviews can be useful decision-making tools for health care consumers and policymakers by objectively summarizing large amounts of information, identifying gaps in medical research, and identifying beneficial or harmful interventions.

- Little published research has evaluated the direct impact of systematic reviews on the health care decisions made by policymakers and consumers.

- Making decisions on health care policies and issues is a complex process in which information, such as that provided by systematic reviews, plays only one part.

- Strategies that increase consumer and policymaker awareness and identification of systematic reviews, that allow critical appraisal of reviews, and that incorporate reviews into the decision-making process should be developed.

- Finding the answers to questions that are relevant to policymakers and consumers requires effective collaboration among medical researchers and other decision makers.

Acknowledgments: The authors thank Gail Kennedy, Stacey Misakian, David Naylor, and Dave Sackett for their useful comments. They also thank the clinical reviewer, Paul F. Speckart.

References

1. **Woolf SH, Battista RN, Anderson GM, Logan AG, Wang E.** Assessing the clinical effectiveness of preventive maneuvers: analytic principles and systematic methods in reviewing evidence and developing clinical practice recommendations. A report by the Canadian Task Force on the Periodic Health Examination. J Clin Epidemiol. 1990;43:891-905.

2. **Diamond GA, Denton TA.** Alternative perspectives on the biased foundations of medical technology assessment. Ann Intern Med. 1993;118:455-64.

3. **Fahey T, Griffiths S, Peters TJ.** Evidence based purchasing: understanding results of clinical trials and systematic reviews. BMJ. 1995;311:1056-9.

4. **Jadad AR.** Are you playing evidence-based medicine games with out daughter? [Letter] Lancet. 1996;347:274.

5. **Light RJ, Pillemer DB.** Summing U p: The Science of Reviewing Research. Cambridge, MA: Harvard Univ Pr; 1984.

6. **Kennedy G, Frockt D, Bero L.** The extend and accuracy of newspaper coverage on environmental tobacco smoke research [Abstract]. American Public Health Association Meeting: New York; 1996.

7. **Weiss C.** Ideology, interests, and information: the basis of policy positions. In: Callahan D, Jennings B, eds. Ethics, The Social Sciences, and Policy Analysis. New York: Plenum; 1983:213-45.

8. **Haynes RB, Sackett DL, Gray JM, Cook DJ, Guyatt GH.** Transferring evidence from research into practice: 1. The role of evidence from clinical care research in clinical decisions [Editorial]. ACP J Club. 1996;125:A14-5.

9. **Rogers EM.** Diffusion of Innovations. 3d ed. New York: Free Pr; 1983.

10. **Bero L.** Executive summary. In: Banta D, Bero L, Bonair A, Cochet C, Espinas J, Freemantle N, eds. Report of the EURASSESS Subgroup on Dissemination and Impact . Stockholm: The Swedish Council on Technology Assessment in Health Care; 1996.

11. **Llewellyn-Thomas HA.** Patients' health-care decision making: a framework for descriptive and experimental investigations. Med Decis Making. 1995;15:101-6.

12. **Solari ME, Wheatley D.** A method of combining the results of several clinical trials. Clin Trials J. 1966;3:537-45.

13. **Cochran WG.** Problems arising in the analysis of a series of similar experiments. Journal of the Royal Statistics Society. 1937;4:102-18.

14. **Yates F, Cochran WG.** The analysis of groups of experiments. J Agric Sci. 1938;28:556-80.

15. **Mulrow CD.** The medical review article: state of the science. Ann Intern Med. 1987;106:485-8.

16. **Bero L, Rennie D.** The Cochrane Collaboration. Preparing, maintaining, and disseminating systematic reviews of the effects of health care. [Editorial]. JAMA. 1995;274:1935-8.

17. **Bucher HC, Schmidt JG.** Does routine ultrasound scanning improve outcome in pregnancy? Meta-analysis of various outcome measures. BMJ. 1996;307:13-7.

18. **Giles W, Bisits A.** Clinical use of Doppler ultrasound in pregnancy: information from six randomised trials. Fetal Diag Ther. 1993;8:247-55.

19. **Neilson J.** Routine ultrasound in early pregnancy. In: Neilson J, Crowther C, Hodnett E, Hofmeyr G, Keirse M, Renfrew M, eds. Pregnancy and Childbirth Module of the Cochrane Database of Systematic Reviews. v 2. London: BMJ Publishing Group; 1996.

20. **Pearson V.** Antenatal ultrasound scanning. Report 26. Bristol, England: Health Care Evaluation Unit, University of Bristol; 1994.

21. **Nisbett R, Ross L.** Improving human inference: possibilities and limitations. In: Nisbett R, Ross L, eds. Human Inference: Strategies and Shortcomings of Social Judgment. Englewood Cliffs, NJ: Prentice-Hall; 1980:273-96.

22. **Glantz SA, Parmley WW.** Passive smoking and heart disease: Epidemiology, physiology, and biochemistry. Circulation. 1991;83:1-12.

23. **Wells AJ.** Passive smoking as a cause of heart disease. J Am Coll Cardiol. 1994;24:546-54.

24. **Steenland K.** Passive smoking and the risk of heart disease. JAMA. 1992;267:94-9.

25. **Cook DJ, Mulrow CD, Haynes RB.** Systematic reviews: synthesis of best evidence for clinical decisions. Ann Intern Med. 1997;128:376-80.

26. **Savulescu J, Chalmers I, Blunt J.** Are research ethics committees behaving unethically? Some suggestions for improving performance and accountability. BMJ. 1996;313:1390-3.

27. **Oliver S, Rajan L, Turner H, Oakley A, Entwistle V, Walt I, et al.** Informed choice for users of health services: views on ultrasonography leaflets of women in early pregnancy, midwives, and ultrasonographers. BMJ. 1996;313:1251-3.

28. **Sullum J, Lieberman B.** Imbalancing act. National Review. 199 5;47:48-52.

29. **Coiera E.** The Internet's challenge to health care provision. A free market in information will conflict with a controlled market in health care. BMJ. 1996;312:3-4.

30. **NHS Executive.** Promoting clinical effectiveness: a framework for action in and through the NHS. United Kingdom: National Health Service, The Department of Health; 1996.

31. **Bastian H.** Finding out what health care works: consumer involvement in research and the Cochrane Collaboration [Editorial]. Health Forum (Journal of the Consumers' Health Forum of Australia). 1994;32:15-6.

32. **Sisk J.** Improving the use of research-based evidence in policy-making: effective care in pregnancy and childbirth in the United States. Milbank Q. 1993;71:477-96.

33. **Greer AL.** The state of the art versus the state of the science. The diffusion of new medical technologies into practice. Int J Technol Assess Health Care. 1988;4:5-26.

34. **Sacks HS, Berrier J, Reitman D, Pagano D, Chalmers TC.** Meta-analysis of randomized controlled trials: an update of the quality and methodology. In: Bailar JC, Mosteller F, eds. Medical Uses of Statistics. 2d ed. Boston: NEJM Books; 1992:427-42.

35. **Jadad AR, McQuay HJ.** Meta-analyses to evaluate analgesic interventions: a systematic qualitative review of their methodology. J Clin Epidemiol. 1996;49:235-43.

36. **The Cochrane Collaboration.** The Cochrane Library [database on disk and CD ROM]. v 2 Oxford: Update Software; 1996 [updated 6 June 1996].

37. **Phillips K, Bero LA.** Improving the use of information in medical effectiveness research. Int J Qual Health Care. 1996;8:21-30.

38. **Barnes D, Bero L.** Quality of Review Articles on Environmental Tobacco Smoke [Abstract]. New York: American Public Health Association Meeting; 1996.

39. **Naylor CD.** Grey zones of clinical practice: some limits to evidence-based medicine. Lancet. 1995;345:840-42.

40. **Redelmeier D, Rozin P, Kahneman D.** Understanding patients' decisions. Cognitive and emotional perspectives. JAMA. 1993;270:72-6.

41. **Goel V, Naylor CD.** Using research and evaluation results in health services policy making. In: Dunn EV, Norton PG, Stewart M, Tudiver F, Bass MJ, eds. Disseminating Research, Changing Practice. v 6. Thousand Oaks: Sage Publications; 1994:199-211.

42. **Dixon A.** The evolution of clinical policies. Med Care. 1990;28:201-20.

43. **Hadorn D, Baker D, Dracup K, Pitt B.** Making judgments about treatment effectiveness based on health outcomes: theoretical and practical issues. Jt Comm J Qual Improv. 1994; 20:547-54.

44. **Goodare H, Smith R.** The rights of patients in research-patients must come first in research. BMJ. 1995;310:1305-6.

45. **Chalmers I.** What do I want from health research and researchers when I am a patient? BMJ. 1995;310:131 5-8.

46. **Jadad AR, Whelan T, Reyno L, et al.** A team approach to pain relief: a guide developed with patients and family members [Abstract]. Supportive Care in Cancer. 1996;3:245.

47. **Scott RA, Shore AR.** Why Sociology Does Not Apply: A Study of the Use of Sociology in Public Planning. New York: Elsevier; 1979.

48. **Jones R, Lamont T, Haines A.** Setting priorities for research and development in the NHS: a case study on the interface between primary and secondary care. BMJ. 1995;311:1076-80.

49. **Oliver SR.** How can health service users contribute to the NHS research and development programme? BMJ. 1995;310:1318-20.

50. **Freemantle N.** Dealing with uncertainty: will science solve the problems of resource allocation in the UK NHS? Soc Sci Med. 1995;40:1365-70.

51. **Caplan N.** What do we know about knowledge utilization? In: Braskamp LA, Brown RD, eds. New Directions for Program Evaluation. San Francisco: Jossey-Bass; 1980.

Chapter 6

The Relation between Systematic Reviews and Practice Guidelines

Deborah J. Cook, MD, MSc(Epid); Nancy L. Greengold, MD;
A. Gray Ellrodt, MD; and Scott R. Weingarten, MD, MPH

Clinical practice guidelines have been developed to improve the process and outcomes of health care and to optimize resource utilization. By addressing such issues as prevention, diagnosis, and treatment, they can aid in health care decision making at many levels. Several other decision aids are cast in the guideline lexicon, regardless of their focus, formulation, or format; this can foster misunderstanding of the term "guideline."

Whether created or adapted locally or nationally, most guidelines are an amalgam of clinical experience, expert opinion, and research evidence. Approaches to practice guideline development vary widely. Given the resources required to identify all relevant primary studies, many guidelines rely on systematic reviews that were either previously published or created *de novo* by guideline developers. Systematic reviews can aid in guideline development because they involve searching for, selecting, critically appraising, and summarizing the results of primary research. The more rigorous the review methods used and the higher the quality of the primary research that is synthesized, the more evidence-based the practice guideline is likely to be. Summaries of relevant research incorporated into guideline documents can help to keep practitioners up to date with the literature. Systematic reviews have also been published on the dissemination and implementation strategies most likely to change clinician behavior and improve patient outcomes. These can be useful in more effectively translating research evidence into practice.

Historically, implicit clinical policies rested primarily with individual practitioners, protected under the rubric of "the art of medicine" and modulated by knowledge, experience, and heuristics (1). Dissemination of information through peer-reviewed publications and traditional continuing medical education represent two major, albeit somewhat passive and indirect, attempts to inform clinical practice. The promulgation of explicit clinical policy embodied in practice guidelines has recently heightened awareness of the determinants of medical decision making (2).

Practice guidelines have been developed to improve the process of health care and health outcomes, decrease practice variation, and optimize resource utilization (3, 4). Described as "systematically developed statements to assist practitioner and patient decisions about appropriate health care for specific clinical circumstances" (5), guidelines attempt to distill a large body of medical expertise into a convenient, readily usable format. Practice guidelines based on the synthesis of the best, most recent evidence can help practitioners keep current with the literature and help them assimilate evidence into practice (6, 7).

The term "guideline" is used loosely to describe documents with different purposes, such as regulation of hospital admissions, use of tests and technology, transfer of seriously ill patients (8), and training programs (9). Sporting such names as "practice policies," "practice parameters," and "clinical indicators" (10, 11), other decision aids further expand this lexicon. Clinical practice guidelines represent specific decision nodes that can be linked together to form clinical pathways or algorithms. Clinical pathways organize, sequence, and time the care given to a "typical, uncomplicated patient" (4, 12), whereas clinical algorithms are a set of more complex instructions for addressing a particular issue in which decisions and their consequences are expressed in conditional, branching logic (13).

This chapter focuses on the relation between systematic reviews and practice guidelines: how the development of guidelines can benefit from systematic reviews, and how systematic reviews can be used to help implement guidelines.

Methods for Developing Guidelines: An Overview

Methods used to develop guidelines differ according to the stakeholders involved, the degree of reliance on formal literature reviews, the extent to which expert opinion prevails, and the process by which the ultimate recommendations are expressed (11). A multidisciplinary team may result in a holistic approach and wider endorsement of the final product (7). Group processes commonly used to generate clinical recommendations include informal peer committees, nominal group techniques (14), the Delphi method (15), and expert or nonexpert consensus conferences. These strategies are not mutually exclusive, and their advantages and disadvantages have been summarized elsewhere (16). One method for guideline development is outlined in Figure 6.1. Whether guidelines are created by local health providers, regional or national professional bodies, payers, or purchasers, the resources available may also determine the focus and methods. Few studies have compared the process, products, and health outcomes of these different approaches to developing recommendations (17).

Selecting the clinical problem to be addressed by a guideline involves considering the prevalence of the problem, the clinical and economic burden it imposes, the resources available for its care, the availability of evidence for both existing care and improved care, and the likelihood of influencing practice (18, 19). The next steps involve learning about current clinical practice as a baseline for change, defining the goals of the guidelines, and searching for the relevant research evidence (Figure 6.1). Because a guideline based on an incomplete or biased evaluation of the literature can lead to inappropriate recommendations, the search for relevant research should be comprehensive, research should be selected by using explicit criteria, and the validity of the results should be judged in a rigorous and reproducible fashion. Guideline and pathway developers ideally search for, select, critique, and combine data in a manner analogous to that used for a systematic review.

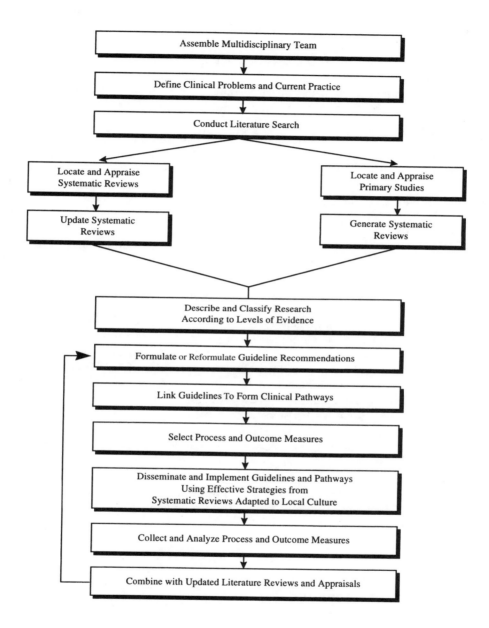

Figure 6.1. One approach to developing guidelines and pathways on the basis of summaries of the relevant research evidence (12). After defining the scope of the guideline and current practice, multidisciplinary teams search for, select, critically appraise, and update published systematic reviews or create their own systematic reviews of the primary literature when none exist (7). The research is then classified according to its rigor, and recommendations are graded accordingly. Systematic reviews are used to select the most effective methods of guideline and pathway implementation, adapted to local circumstances. Updated systematic reviews, lessons learned through the implementation experience, and analysis of process measures and clinical and economic outcomes are then used to reformulate guidelines and pathways as a method of continuous quality improvement.

In addition to incorporating evidence and acknowledging its absence, creating clinical recommendations requires making value judgments about preferred courses of action. Some guidelines lay out choices and are distinctively influenced by patient preferences. Consider the difference in this regard between offering men with prostate cancer the choice of conservative management or radical prostatectomy (which builds patient preference into the decision) and assuming that all patients without advance directives who sustain a cardiac arrest want cardiopulmonary resuscitation (which does not).

Guideline documents ideally indicate how disagreements were handled and how information was synthesized (for example, by a qualitative pooling of opinion, a quantitative approach such as meta-analysis or decision analysis, or some combination of methods [19]). If guideline developers do not indicate how they identified and summarized the evidence and integrated different values, clinicians cannot adequately evaluate the rigor of the guidelines and the extent to which research evidence supports the recommendations (20, 21). Recent guidelines for the diagnosis and treatment of idiopathic thrombocytopenic purpura (22) described the literature, emphasized the paucity of evidence and the limitations of opinion-based recommendations, and issued recommendations on the basis of clear documentation of the strength and variance of opinion (23).

The Role of Research Evidence in Practice Guideline Development

Guideline developers who want to incorporate research evidence into their clinical recommendations recognize the challenges of exhaustively searching the literature. For many common conditions, the volume of clinically useful literature is considerable. For other conditions, data may be sparse. Because guideline development is often limited by the difficulty of locating and appraising primary research, searching for and conducting systematic reviews is important. Accordingly, both primary research and integrative articles are potentially useful to guideline developers (Figure 6.1).

Systematic reviews are the most common type of integrative article. Their authors have searched for, selected, and synthesized (either qualitatively or quantitatively) evidence on specific clinical questions. Economic analyses quantitatively compare the costs and consequences of alternate courses of action. Decision analyses present the probability of various outcomes in terms of the values of expected benefits and harms of key decisions. Although clinical recommendations may emerge from these documents, their content is typically structured in a research report format. In contrast, practice guidelines are more often presented in a framework congruent with decision making; they suggest or support specific clinical recommendations but may reflect the scope of information contained in systematic reviews, economic analyses, and decision analyses.

For example, the American College of Physicians guidelines for magnetic resonance imaging of the brain and spine (24) were produced after a systematic review of neuroimaging with magnetic resonance imaging (25), and the guideline developers acknowledged the absence of studies comparing magnetic resonance imaging with other technologies. Relevant reviews are sometimes published after rather than before guidelines are developed. Such was the case with the 1994 clinical practice guideline on unstable angina by the Agency for Health Care Policy and Research (26), whose expert panel recommended that patients with unstable angina who are receiving aspirin should be treated with heparin for 2 to 5 days unless heparin is contraindicated. Two years later, a supporting meta-analysis showed a 33% reduction in risk for myocardial infarction or death in patients who had unstable angina and received aspirin plus heparin compared with those who received aspirin alone (27).

The scope of guidelines may reflect the particular interests of the guideline developers. The College's guidelines for the medical treatment of stroke prevention (28) clearly incorporate the results of a concurrently published systematic review (29) but are not explicit about cost-effectiveness issues (such as the rationale for choosing aspirin rather than ticlopidine). Other guidelines, such as those created by the American Heart Association for carotid endarterectomy (30), comprehensively summarize research and address economic issues more directly.

Examples of How To Use Systematic Reviews for Building Practice Guidelines and Clinical Pathways

As an alternate or complementary approach to formally summarizing primary research, guideline and pathway developers can use previously published systematic reviews that summarize the relevant primary studies. For the management of bleeding esophageal varices, approximately 200 randomized trials of pharmacologic, mechanical, and surgical interventions could be considered, as could a more manageable number of systematic reviews of these topics. For example, systematic reviews of primary prevention of variceal gastrointestinal hemorrhage indicate that β-blockade and sclerotherapy reduce bleeding and mortality rates (31-33). Systematic reviews also indicate the following. First, for control of acute bleeding, vasopressin is superior to no treatment but somatostatin is more effective than vasopressin (34, 35).

Second, although emergency sclerotherapy controls bleeding and decreases rebleeding rates more than do drug treatment and balloon tamponade (35), ligation is more effective than sclerotherapy (36). Third, for the prevention of rebleeding, both sclerotherapy and β-blockade are beneficial, but they are more effective in combination than either one is alone (35). Finally, although shunt surgery decreases the risk for bleeding when performed prophylactically and decreases the risk for rebleeding when done as treatment, surgery markedly increases the risk for hepatic encephalopathy and may hasten death in both settings (35). In summary, persons developing clinical pathways who are interested in the broad spectrum of decisions associated with long-term management of variceal bleeding have a solid database of well-conducted systematic reviews of rigorous trials on which to build.

A focused initiative based on results of one systematic review might involve the creation of a single guideline. Investigators at Cedars-Sinai Medical Center in Los Angeles, for example, concentrated on early endoscopy and a short hospital stay for certain "low-risk" patients with nonvariceal gastrointestinal hemorrhage. A systematic review indicated that early therapeutic endoscopy has a favorable effect on rebleeding, surgery, and mortality (37), suggesting that timely risk stratification and treatment chosen according to clinical and endoscopic features would allow clinicians to consider early discharge of patients at low risk for adverse events. The promising results of a retrospective validation study that examined the effect of a guideline recommending this approach (38) were confirmed by a prospective time series study. This study showed that management of patients in accordance with the guideline resulted in no difference in morbidity or mortality but led to greater patient satisfaction, shorter hospital stays, and lower costs (39).

Limitations of Relying on Systematic Reviews in Guideline Development

Although systematic reviews of treatment can lay the foundation for practice guidelines, they are not a panacea. The most fundamental limitation of relying on reviews is that they never obviate the need for at least some critical appraisal of the original studies to understand the populations, interventions, and outcomes evaluated; the heterogeneity of these features; and the individual study results.

Considering our variceal bleeding example, trials of new treatment (for example, octreotide after variceal ligation [40] and combination β-blocker and nitrate therapy [41]), as well as new surgical interventions, such as transjugular intrahepatic portosystemic shunting and liver transplantation (42), may not be summarized in systematic reviews. Even if guidelines are based on a careful systematic review of one approach (such as medical prevention of strokes [28]), the final recommendations may be narrowly focused (for example, by not considering carotid endarterectomy).

Not all outcomes of interest are measured in all primary studies; thus, certain measures, such as quality of life, are often inadequately represented in reviews. Because most randomized trials are underpowered for rare events or unusual adverse effects of treatment and may not report them, systematic reviews do not usually provide such information. Making diagnoses, triaging, and understanding patient preferences require alternate study designs; such material is less likely to be summarized in systematic reviews. The same holds for many other aspects of clinical practice based on pathophysiologic rationale and conventional wisdom. Obviously, sole reliance on systematic reviews will never adequately serve development of guidelines and pathways.

Systematic reviews and, therefore, the practice guidelines based on them may require modification in areas for which evidence continually emerges. For example, the results of a 1985 systematic review of randomized trials suggesting that histamine-2-receptor antagonists were beneficial in acute nonvariceal gastrointestinal bleeding (43) were questioned 7 years later by a large, more rigorous negative trial of a newer histamine-2-receptor antagonist, famotidine (44). The postulate that acid suppression averts rebleeding was further challenged by another large negative trial of the proton pump inhibitor omeprazole (45); this trial showed that the drug had no benefit in terms of rebleeding, need for surgery, or mortality. Emphasizing the vicissitudes of this situation is the most recent trial of high-dose oral omeprazole, which decreased continued or further bleeding and surgery in patients with ulcer (46).

Examining published reviews (and the primary research these reviews summarize) in preparation for guideline formulation often shows that research is insufficient to inform management decisions. Exposing gaps in medical knowledge can be a powerful stimulus for future research by guideline developers.

Finally, as the number of systematic reviews continues to increase, clinicians will be increasingly faced with more than one review on the same topic. Such multiple reviews may be helpful, particularly if later reviews update earlier ones, if one review resolves disagreements among previous reviews (47), or if concurrently published reviews yield concordant results. However, multiple systematic reviews may also challenge guideline and pathway developers if they generate conflicting conclusions. Strategies for dealing with such situations include careful critical appraisal of each review (48), with particular emphasis on issues of clinical and statistical heterogeneity (49), and a more detailed assessment of the relation between the focus of each review and the specific purpose of the guideline under development.

Using Systematic Reviews for the Format and Expression of Guidelines

To maximize the chance that guidelines reach the right practitioners at the right time and to help practitioners make the right decisions for the right patients, guidelines should be available at the place and time of decision making. Clinicians prefer short manuals or summaries of major recommendations and a synopsis of the underlying evidence that summarizes expected benefits and harms (50). Publication of companion systematic reviews and executive summaries of their results may therefore be useful in guideline dissemination. Embedding guidelines in electronic medical records may also be helpful.

The strength of treatment recommendations is ideally informed by the quality of the research evidence; the magnitude, precision, and reproducibility of the treatment effect; and the relative value (determined by guideline developers, health care workers, and patients) of various outcomes. A key component of guidelines, therefore, is how accurately they reflect the inference conferred by the underlying research evidence. When all else is equal, recommendations about therapy are strongest when they are derived from systematic reviews of randomized trials that have consistent results, as opposed to reviews of trials or observational studies that have inconsistent results (51).

For example, the American College of Chest Physicians Antithrombotic Consensus Conferences classify evidence as level I (evidence obtained from randomized trials or meta-analyses of randomized trials, for which the lower limit of the CI around the point estimate of the treatment effect exceeds the minimal clinically important benefit), level II (evidence obtained from randomized trials or meta-analyses, for which the lower level of the CI around the treatment effect overlaps the minimal clinically important benefit), level III (evidence obtained from nonrandomized, concurrent cohort studies), level IV (evidence obtained from nonrandomized historical cohort studies), and level V (evidence obtained from case series or expert opinion) (52). Thus, for example, the American College of Chest Physicians assigned a grade C recommendation to the use of long-term anticoagulation in patients with bioprosthetic valves and a history of systemic embolism; this grade is based on the use of level V evidence (expert opinion) in the formulation of the recommendations (53). In this way, guidelines can avoid ambiguous terminology because readers are made aware of the basis for the recommendations and the extent to which the recommendations reflect the strength of the research evidence (Figure 6.1).

Using Systematic Reviews of Implementation Strategies for Practice Guidelines

Because the construction of guidelines alone does not change clinical practice, the next step is to disseminate and implement them (Figure 6.1). Some modern guideline documents describe how the guidelines were developed, but they rarely contain information on dissemination and implementation strategies. As described below, several systematic reviews (54-57) have summarized the studies that sought to determine which methods are most effective for changing clinician behavior and patient health status. Modification of provider practices and other "process measures" have been the outcomes most often studied. Although these may be viewed as less important surrogate outcomes, if selected carefully they can be viewed as intermediate steps that causally link recommendations to more meaningful patient-centered outcomes.

A systematic review of 59 rigorous studies evaluating the effect of practice guidelines found that 55 of them detected significant improvements in the process of care after introduction of the guidelines (54). An update of this review (55) indicated that 12 of 17 studies assessing patient outcome after guideline implementation reported significant improvement in at least one outcome. Several insights emerged from this work. For example, the most effective strategies for implementing practice guidelines are educational interventions that are developed within local organizations and implemented through patient-specific reminders, whereas the least effective are externally developed guidelines that are disseminated through publications and implemented by general reminders.

These findings complement data summarized in another review of educational interventions targeted at changing the performance of practicing physicians and the health of their patients. Davis and colleagues (56) examined 99 randomized trials of continuing medical education. Almost two thirds of the trials showed an improvement in at least one outcome; 70% showed a change in physician behavior, and 48% of interventions aimed at health outcomes produced a positive change. Effective strategies included specific reminders, patient-mediated interventions, outreach visits (including academic detailing and opinion leaders), and other multifaceted activities. Formal continuing medical education sessions without practice-reinforcing strategies, educational materials, and audit and feedback were not found to be very effective. Another systematic review of the controlled studies evaluating computer-based clinical decision support systems showed that clinician behavior and patient outcomes can be modified by the use of these methods (57).

The less compelling the research evidence incorporated into guidelines, the greater is the need to test the impact of the guidelines on patient outcomes. Therefore, rigorous evaluation depends on understanding not just the guideline development process but also the specific methods used to disseminate and implement the guidelines. To date, systematic reviews have summarized single and multiple implementation methods. Although complex, multimethod approaches are frequently used, current knowledge of their effectiveness and generalizability remains somewhat limited. In making such evaluations, it is important to consider the health care setting in which the guidelines are implemented; valid practice guidelines coupled with effective implementation strategies may have no impact if constraints of access, availability, or cost are very strong or if attitudinal barriers prevent their endorsement (58). Moreover, no matter how they are developed and implemented, guidelines may do more harm than good if they are inappropriately interpreted or applied.

Summary

In the past decade, the practice guidelines movement has become a major academic and commercial enterprise. If created by using the most valid and current research evidence summarized in systematic reviews, guidelines are one of many tools that can help to translate research evidence into clinical decision aids, optimize health outcomes, and educate clinicians. Like all decision aids, however, guidelines should be integrated with pathophysiologic reasoning and experience and should be adopted, adapted, or rejected according to patient preferences and the constraints of each health care setting. Practice guidelines and clinical pathways have potential limitations, many of which can be overcome by using an evidence-based approach in their development and by drawing on state-of-the-art implementation strategies that themselves have been summarized in systematic reviews. This field is ripe for future health services research.

Key Points To Remember

- Formal reviews of the literature are fundamental to the development of sound practice guidelines.

- Developers of evidence-based guidelines generate their own systematic reviews and critically appraise and update previously published systematic reviews.

- When current systematic reviews are presented as companion documents to practice guidelines, they can help to communicate the evidence that supports specific clinical recommendations.

- Like all research evidence, data summarized in systematic reviews are important but not sufficient for practice guideline development; accordingly, recommendations should be interpreted in light of patient preferences and the health care setting in which the recommendations are implemented, which governs issues of feasibility and finance.

- Systematic reviews of the effectiveness of strategies for disseminating and implementing guidelines can be used to help select the approach that will produce the maximum impact on caregiver behavior and patient outcome.

Acknowledgments: The authors thank Dr. Walter Peterson for his helpful suggestions. They also thank the clinical reviewer, Paul Speckart.

References

1. **McDonald CJ.** Medical heuristics: the silent adjudicators of clinical practice. Ann Intern Med. 1996;124:56-62.
2. **Lomas J.** Making clinical policy explicit. Legislative policy making and lessons for developing practice guidelines. Int J Technol Assess Health Care. 1993;9:11-25.
3. **Audet AM, Greenfield S, Field M.** Medical practice guidelines: current activities and future directions. Ann Intern Med. 1990;113:709-14.
4. **Pearson SD, Goulart-Fisher D, Lee TH.** Critical pathways as a strategy for improving care: problems and potential. Ann Intern Med. 1995;123:941-8.
5. **Field MJ, Lohr KN.** Clinical Practice Guidelines: Directions of a New Program. Washington, DC: National Academy Pr; 1990.
6. **Handley MR, Stuart ME.** An evidence-based approach to evaluating and improving clinical practice guideline development. HMO Practice. 1994;10-9.
7. **Greengold NL, Weingarten SR.** Developing evidence-based practice guidelines and pathways: the experience at the local hospital level. Jt Comm J Qual Improv. 1996;22:391-402.
8. Guidelines for the transfer of critically ill patients. Guidelines Committee of the American College of Critical Care Medicine; Society of Critical Care Medicine and American Association of Critical-Care Nurses Transfer Guidelines Task Force. Crit Care Med. 1993;21:931-7.
9. Guidelines for a training programme in intensive care medicine. European Society of Intensive Care Medicine, European Society of Pediatric Intensive Care. Intensive Care Med. 1996;22:166-72.
10. **Eddy DM.** Clinical decision making: from theory to practice. Practice policies-what are they? JAMA. 1990;263:877-8.
11. **Woolf SH.** Practice guidelines: A new reality in medicine. I. Recent developments. Arch Intern Med. 1990;150:1811-8.
12. **Deignan M, Ellrodt AG.** Resource management. In: Aydin CE, Bolton LB, Weingarten S, eds. Patient-focused Care in the Hospital: Restructuring and Redesign Methods to Achieve Better Outcomes. New York: Faulkner & Gray; 1995.
13. **Schoenbaum SC, ed.** Using Clinical Practice Guidelines to Evaluate Quality of Care. v 1. Bethesda, MD: U.S. Department of Health and Human Services; 1995. AHCPR publication no. 95-0045.
14. **Fink A, Kosecoff J, Chassin M, Brook RH.** Consensus methods: characteristics and guidelines for use. Am J Public Health. 1984;74:979-83.
15. **Dalkey NC.** The Delphi method: an experimental study of group opinion. Santa Monica, CA: RAND Corp.; 1969. Publication no. RM-58888 PR.
16. **Woolf SH.** Practice guidelines: a new reality in medicine. II. Methods of developing guidelines. Arch Intern Med. 1992;152:946-52.
17. **Lomas J.** Words without action? The production, dissemination, and impact of consensus recommendations. Annu Rev Public Health. 1991;12:41-65.
18. **Browman GP, Levine MN, Mohide A, Hayward RS, Pritchard KI, Gafni A, et al.** The practice guidelines development cycle: a conceptual tool for practice guidelines development and implementation. J Clin Oncol. 1995;13:502-12.
19. **Hayward RS, Laupacis A.** Initiating, conducting and maintaining guidelines development programs. Can Med Assoc J. 1993;148:507-12.
20. **Hayward RS, Wilson MC, Tunis SR, Bass EB, Guyatt GH.** Users' guides to the medical literature. VIII. How to use clinical practice guidelines. A. Are the recommendations valid? The Evidence-Based Medicine Working Group. JAMA. 1995;274:570-4.
21. **Wilson MC, Hayward RS, Tunis SR, Bass EB, Guyatt GH.** Users' guides to the medical litera-

ture. VIII. How to use clinical practice guidelines. B. What are the recommendations and will they help you in caring for your patients? The Evidence-Based Medicine Working Group. JAMA. 1995;274:1630-2.

22. **George FN, Davidoff F.** Idiopathic thrombocytopenic purpura: lessons from a guideline. Ann Intern Med. 1997;126:317-8.

23. Diagnosis and treatment of idiopathic thrombocytopenic purpura: recommendations of the American Society of Hematology. The American Society of Hematology ITP Practice Guideline Panel. Ann Intern Med. 1997;126:319-26.

24. **American College of Physicians.** Magnetic resonance imaging of the brain and spine: a revised statement. Ann Intern Med. 1994;120:872-5.

25. **Kent DL, Haynor DR, Longstreth WT Jr, Larson EB.** The clinical efficacy of magnetic resonance imaging in neuroimaging. Ann Intern Med. 1994;120:856-75.

26. **Crawford MH.** Unstable angina: diagnosis and management. Clinical practice guidelines no. 10. New York: Chapman & Hall; 1997.

27. **Oler A, Whooley MA, Oler J, Grady D.** Adding heparin to aspirin reduces the incidence of myocardial infarction and death in patients with unstable angina. A meta-analysis. JAMA. 1966; 276:811-5.

28. **American College of Physicians.** Guidelines for medical treatment for stroke prevention. Ann Intern Med. 1994;121:54-5.

29. **Matchar DB, McCrory DC, Barnett HJ, Feussner JR.** Medical treatment for stroke prevention. Ann Intern Med. 1994;121:41-53.

30. **Moore WS, Barnett HJ, Beebe HG, Bernstein EF, Brener BJ, Brott T, et al.** Guidelines for carotid endarterectomy: a multidisciplinary consensus statement from the Ad Hoc Committee, American Heart Association. Circulation. 1995;91: 566-79.

31. **Van Ruiswyk J, Byrd JC.** Efficacy of prophylactic sclerotherapy for the prevention of a first variceal hemorrhage. Gastroenterology. 1992;102: 587-97.

32. **Pagliaro L, D'Amico G, Sorensen TI, Lebrec D, Burroughs AK, Morabito A, et al.** Prevention of first bleeding in cirrhosis. A meta-analysis of randomized trials of nonsurgical treatment. Ann Intern Med. 1992;117:59-70.

33. **Fardy JM, Laupacis A.** A meta-analysis of prophylactic endoscopic sclerotherapy for esophageal varices. Am J Gastroenterol. 1994;89:1938-48.

34. **Gotzsche PC, Gjorup I, Bonnen H, Brahe NE, Becker U, Burcharth F.** Somatostatin v placebo in bleeding oesophageal varices: randomised trial and meta-analysis. BMJ. 1995;310:1495-8.

35. **D'Amico G, Pagliaro L, Bosch J.** The treatment of portal hypertension: a meta-analytic review. Hepatology. 1995;22:332-54.

36. **Laine L, Cook D.** Endoscopic ligation compared with sclerotherapy for treatment of esophageal variceal bleeding. A meta-analysis. Ann Intern Med. 1995;123:280-7.

37. **Cook DJ, Guyatt GH, Salena BJ, Laine LA.** Endoscopic therapy for acute nonvariceal upper gastrointestinal hemorrhage: a meta-analysis. Gastroenterology. 1992;102:139-48.

38. **Hay JA, Lyubashevsky E, Elashoff J, Maldonado L, Weingarten SR, Ellrodt AG.** Upper gastrointestinal hemorrhage clinical guideline-determining the optimal hospital length of stay. Am J Med. 1996;100:313-22.

39. **Hay JA, Ellrodt AG, Weingarten SR.** Prospective validation of a length-of-stay guideline for upper gastrointestinal hemorrhage. Am J Gastroenterol. 1995;90:1661.

40. **Sung JJ, Chung SC, Yung MY, Lai CW, Lau JY, Lee YT, et al.** Prospective randomised study of effect of octreotide on rebleeding from oesophageal varices after endoscopic ligation. Lancet. 1995;346:1666-9.

41. **Villanueva C, Balanzo J, Novella MT, Soriano G, Sainz S, Torras X, et al.** Nadolol plus isosorbide mononitrate compared with sclerotherapy for the prevention of variceal bleeding. N Engl J Med. 1996;334:1624-9.

42. **Cello JP, Ring EJ, Olcott EW, Koch J, Gordon R.** Endoscopic sclerotherapy compared with percutaneous transjugular intrahepatic portosystemic shunt after initial sclerotherapy in patients with acute variceal hemorrhage. A randomized, controlled trial. Ann Intern Med. 1997;126:858-65.

43. **Collins R, Langman M.** Treatment with histamine H2 antagonists in acute upper gastrointestinal hemorrhage. Implications of randomized trials. N Engl J Med. 1985;313:660-6.

44. **Walt RP, Cottrell J, Mann SG, Freemantle NP, Langman MJ.** Continuous intravenous famotidine for haemorrhage from peptic ulcer. Lancet. 1992;340:1058-62.

45. **Daneshmend TK, Hawkey CJ, Langman MJ, Logan RF, Long RG, Walt RP, et al.** Omeprazole versus placebo for acute upper gastrointestinal bleeding: randomised double blind controlled trial. BMJ. 1992;304:143-7.

46. **Khuroo MS, Yattoo GN, Javid G, Khan BA, Shah AA, Gulzar GM, et al.** A comparison of omeprazole and placebo for bleeding peptic ulcer. N Engl J Med. 1997;336:1054-8.

47. **Cook DJ, Reeve BK, Guyatt GH, Heyland DK, Griffith LE, Buckingham L, et al.** Stress ulcer prophylaxis in critically ill patients. Resolving discordant meta-analyses. JAMA. 1996;275:308-14.

48. **Oxman AD, Cook DJ, Guyatt GH.** Users' guides to the medical literature. VI. How to use an overview. Evidence-Based Medicine Working Group. JAMA. 1994;272:1367-71.

49. **Jadad A, Cook DJ, Browman G.** When arbitrators disagree: resolving discordant meta-analysis. Can Med Assoc J. 1997;156:141-6.

50. **Hayward RS, Wilson MC, Tunis SR, Guyatt GH, Moore KA, Bass EB.** Practice guidelines. What are internists looking for? J Gen Intern Med. 1996;11:176-8.

51. **Guyatt GH, Sackett DL, Sinclair JC, Hayward R, Cook DJ, Cook RJ.** Users' guides to the medical literature. IX. A method for grading health

care recommendations. Evidence-Based Medicine Working Group. JAMA. 1995;274:1800-4.

52. **Cook DJ, Guyatt GH, Laupacis A, Sackett DL, Goldberg RJ.** Clinical recommendations using levels of evidence for antithrombotic agents. Chest. 1995;108:227S-230S.

53. **Stein PD, Alpert JS, Copeland J, Dalen JE, Goldman S, Turpie AG.** Antithrombotic therapy in patients with mechanical and biologic prosthetic heart valves. Chest. 1995;108:371S-379S.

54. **Grimshaw JM, Russell IT.** Effect of clinical guidelines on medical practice: a systematic review of rigorous evaluations. Lancet. 1993;342:1317-22.

55. **Grimshaw J, Freemantle N, Wallace S, Russell I, Hurwitz B, Watt I, et al.** Developing and implementing clinical practice guidelines. Qual Health Care. 1995;4:55-64.

56. **Davis DA, Thomson MA, Oxman AD, Haynes RB.** Changing physician performance. A systematic review of the effect of continuing medical educational strategies. JAMA. 1995;274:700-5.

57. **Johnston ME, Langton KB, Haynes RB, Mathieu A.** Effects of computer-based clinical decision support systems on clinical performance and patient outcome. A critical appraisal of research. Ann Intern Med. 1994;120:135-42.

58. **Tunis SR, Hayward RS, Wilson MC, Rubin HR, Bass EB, Johnston M, et al.** Internists' attitudes about clinical practice guidelines. Ann Intern Med. 1994;120:956-63.

Chapter 7

Formulating Questions and Locating Primary Studies for Inclusion in Systematic Reviews

Carl Counsell, MRCP(UK)

Much time and effort are spent on designing primary research studies. Similar care must be given to planning systematic reviews. The review should be based on an important, well-focused question that is relevant to patient care. By formulating the question properly, the criteria that primary studies must meet to be included in the review become clear. These criteria, which comprise the types of persons involved, exposure, control group, outcomes, and study designs of interest, can then be refined so that they are clinically relevant, sensible, and workable. Inclusion criteria that are too narrow will limit the amount of data in the review, thereby increasing the risk for chance results and making the review less useful for the reader. Reviews should include studies whose designs offer the least biased answer to the question being asked. To maximize available data and reduce the risk for bias, as many relevant studies as possible need to be identified, regardless of publication status or language. Multiple overlapping search strategies should therefore be used and must be carefully planned. Strategies include searching the many electronic databases available (after careful consideration of which terms to enter), manually searching journals and conference proceedings, searching bibliographies of articles, searching existing registers of studies, and contacting companies or researchers. The time taken to formulate the question adequately and develop appropriate searches will increase the chance of producing a high-quality, meaningful review.

A good systematic review is based on a well-formulated, answerable question. The question guides the review by defining which studies will be included, what the search strategy to identify the relevant primary studies should be, and which data need to be extracted from each study. Ask a poor question and you will get a poor review. A clear question also helps the reader rapidly assess whether the review is relevant to his or her own clinical practice. I discuss where good questions come from, how to choose an important question, how to formulate the question properly to get an answer with an appropriate level of detail, and how to develop a search strategy to identify relevant studies.

Where Do Questions Come From?

Questions arise constantly in routine clinical practice, provided that clinicians are prepared to admit their own level of uncertainty or lack of knowledge (1). The most relevant questions are often asked directly or indirectly by patients (2, 3). Most clinical encounters generate questions about diagnosis ("What do I have, doctor?"), etiology ("Is it because I did X?"), prognosis ("How long do I have?"), or treatment or prevention ("Will Y do me any good?"). The ways in which different clinicians manage the same clinical problem vary widely, both within and between countries; these variations should raise questions about which management policies are best. The introduction of new treatments or diagnostic tests should always lead to the question, "Are they better than what we have already?" Researchers who are planning new studies must consider whether the answer to their question already exists, whereas purchasers of health care must ask which health care packages they should buy. Systematic reviews of all available information would help in each of these situations.

Choosing an Important Question

The number of possible questions for systematic reviews is limitless, but the time and resources with which to answer them are limited. Therefore, researchers who undertake systematic reviews must choose the most important questions. This is difficult because the importance of a question varies according to the perspective of the person asking it. For example, individual patients will probably regard questions about their conditions as the most impor-

tant, regardless of how common or severe that condition is, whereas cardiologists will prefer questions about ischemic heart disease to those about migraine. Cancer and vascular disease are particularly important to persons in developed countries, whereas infectious diseases are more important to persons in developing countries. These differences highlight the need for each specialty to organize its own systematic reviews. Several factors should be considered when setting priorities for doing systematic reviews (4-8) (Table 7.1).

Important questions may deal with conditions that have a major effect on patients or on persons who care for them, such as conditions associated with serious illness (diabetes), death (cancer), or with impaired quality of life (back pain). Very common conditions may have a major effect on society even if they are minor and short-lived (such as the common cold, which results in many aggregate days of missed work). Most health care interventions have potentially harmful effects and should be carefully evaluated. It is particularly important to assess expensive interventions (for example, interferon therapy for multiple sclerosis [9]); widely used interventions, because these may cause widespread harm (for example, lignocaine in acute myocardial infarction [10]); and simple interventions that could be widely used if they are shown to be effective (such as steroids for preterm delivery [11]).

The most useful reviews are those that can improve clinical practice. Widespread change is more likely to occur if collective uncertainty exists; this uncertainty is often reflected in variations in practice. Asking a question that has already been answered by common sense or by powerful empirical evidence is of little use unless evidence suggests that the existing answer is wrong. It is also difficult to influence well-established practices, even if the evidence for their utility is poor (for example, cervical screening programs); new technologies

Table 7.1   Factors To Consider When Determining the Importance of a Question as the Basis for a
Systematic Review

Disease or Condition	Intervention	Ability To Change Practice	Feasibility of Assessment	Other
Effect on the patient or caregiver	Frequency of use or potential for use	Uncertainty of benefit or variation in practice	Availability of data	Interest and enthusiasm of reviewers
Severity (mortality, morbidity, quality of life)				
Duration				
Financial cost (such as loss of earnings)				
Effect on society	Financial cost	Degree of established preferences	Financial cost	Degree of innovativeness
Prevalence				
Severity				
Financial cost (such as lost production)		Timing (such as time since introduction of new practice or technology		Topicality
		Motivation to change		Ethical, social, and political considerations

must therefore be assessed early in their development. Some researchers consider it more important to concentrate on questions for which data are known to exist (4, 5), but this reasoning may be flawed. A thorough search often identifies previously unknown data or a lack of useful data for some important questions, thereby demonstrating the need for future research.

Although the factors in Table 7.1 primarily concern the assessment of health technology, most also apply to prioritizing questions about risk or prognostic factors (that is, the frequency, reversibility, and measurability of the factors). Clearly, many of the factors are relatively subjective (such as effect on the patient), thereby underscoring the need to involve patients in setting priorities (2, 3).

Formulating the Question

Having decided that a question is worth asking, the next step is to formulate it adequately (Figure 7.1). Clinical questions should have four basic components (12): the type of person involved, the type of

exposure that the person experiences (be it a risk factor, a prognostic factor, an intervention, or a diagnostic test), the type of control with which the exposure is being compared, and the outcomes to be addressed.

A clearly formulated question helps define the criteria that studies must meet to be included in the review (Figure 7.2). These inclusion criteria can be divided into five categories, shown in Table 7.2. Each component must be carefully defined to strike a balance between making the definition too specific to be workable and making it too broad to be useful. In Figure 7.2, the definition of *ischemic stroke* could be "a stroke with an occluded artery on angiography"; this definition, however, would exclude most studies because few patients with stroke undergo angiography. Alternatively, it could be defined simply as "ischemic cerebrovascular disease," but it then becomes unclear whether patients with transient ischemic attacks and vascular dementia are included. Some complex exposures or interventions can be difficult to define precisely, especially if they are

Table 7.2   Categories of Inclusion Criteria

Type of person

Disease or condition

  Definition

  Cause

  Stage

  Severity

Personal characteristics

  Age

  Sex

  Symptoms

Population or setting

  Community

  Hospital (outpatient or inpatient)

Type of exposure

Definition

Intensity or dose

Timing

Duration

Method of delivery (group therapy or individual therapy, oral therapy or intravenous therapy)

Type of control

Absence of risk or prognostic factor (risk and prognostic reviews)

Gold standard test (diagnostic reviews)

Treatment controls (treatment and prevention reviews)

  Active treatment or no treatment

  Placebo control or open control

Type of outcome

Importance to patient

  Clinically relevant or surrogate

  Death, quality of life, disability, and symptoms or signs

Beneficial and harmful effects of interventions

Use of health care resources (economic evaluations)

Definitions

Timing of outcome assessment

Type of study design

Experimental or observational

Randomized or nonrandomized controlled trials

Blinded or open trials

Confounded or unconfounded studies (that is, in a comparison of treatment A versus no treatment, a trial of treatment A and treatment B versus no treatment is confounded by treatment B, whereas a trial of A and B versus B alone is not confounded)

nonpharmacologic (for example, how does one define speech therapy?). In this situation, it may be useful to begin with a broad working definition that can later be refined and to test the reproducibility of the definition among different types of persons (for example, *speech therapy* could be defined as "therapy given by a qualified speech therapist to improve language function"). It is also important to remember that definitions may vary among countries and among studies (for example, the term *chronic cerebrovascular disease* is sometimes used to mean "vascular dementia").

The outcomes to be assessed should be clinically relevant to the patient (13). They must consider the perspective of the patient because physicians and patients often do not agree on what issues are important (2, 3). Indirect or surrogate outcome measures, such as laboratory or radiologic results, should be avoided or interpreted with extreme caution because they rarely predict clinically important outcomes accurately (14). Surrogate measures may tell you how a treatment might work but not whether it actually does work. Many treatments reduce the risk for a surrogate outcome but have no effect or have harmful effects on clinically relevant outcomes, and some treatments have no effect on surrogate measures but improve clinical outcomes (14). For example, lignocaine has been shown to suppress ventricular arrhythmias after myocardial infarction (15) but increases case-fatality rates (10). Systematic reviews of treatments should measure adverse effects as well as beneficial effects. Reviewers may also wish to record data on costs to perform an economic evaluation, although this requires expert guidance (16). In addition to defining the outcomes that are to be measured, the inclusion criteria must state when the outcomes should be measured. For chronic diseases, outcomes

A Poorly Formulated Question

Are **anticoagulant agents** useful in **patients who have had stroke**?

A Well-Formulated Question

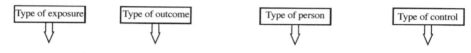

Do **anticoagulant agents** improve **outcomes** in patients with **acute ischemic stroke** compared with **no treatment**?

Figure 7.1 Examples of poorly formulated and well-formulated questions.

that are assessed after a short follow-up period may not reflect long-term outcome.

Reviews should always focus on the best available evidence: that is, studies to be included in a review should use methods that provide the least biased answer to the question asked. Therefore, systematic reviews of treatment and prevention should include randomized, controlled trials (17), particularly those that use a well-concealed method of allocation (18). Reviews of diagnostic tests should include studies that independently compared one or more tests with an adequate gold standard (19, 20). Reviews of prognosis should include cohort studies in which a representative sample of patients was entered at a similar point in the course of disease (21). Finally, reviews of risk factors could include relevant case-control, cohort, or ecologic studies, ideally with multivariate analysis to adjust for other known risk factors. If no studies providing the best level of evidence are found, it may be appropriate to consider other levels of evidence. For example, no evidence from randomized, controlled trials suggests that lying babies supine rather than prone prevents the sudden infant death syndrome,

but a substantial body of observational data suggests that this is the case (22). Other details that must be considered are the requirement for blinding in randomized, controlled trials (18) and studies of diagnostic tests (19, 20) and the presence of confounding factors (Table 7.2).

How Broad Should the Inclusion Criteria Be?

The scope of the question and, hence, the inclusion criteria can be relatively broad or narrow. The choice of inclusion criteria depends on several factors. Questions must be clinically relevant: A broad question ("Has chemotherapy improved cancer survival?") will not help a clinician manage a patient with a particular tumor because of marked differences in the responses of different tumors. Inclusion criteria must also be clinically sensible. If certain features of the patients or exposures are believed to significantly affect outcome, these features must be taken into account. For example, the effects of anticoagulation therapy will probably differ in patients with hemorrhagic stroke compared with patients with ischemic stroke; thus, it is sensible to restrict the question in Figure 7.2 to ischemic strokes. However, narrow inclusion criteria limit the amount of data in the review and thereby increase the risk for false-positive and false-negative results (23, 24). A narrow question can be regarded as a subgroup of a broader question and can lead to the same problems generally found in subgroup analysis (25, 26). Narrow inclusion criteria also preclude studying appropriate and clinically important subgroups in the context of a larger data set. A review of the effects of 5000 units of unfractionated heparin given twice daily in acute stroke will not allow comparisons of the effects of different anticoagulant agents or different doses of heparin. Broad inclusion criteria increase the risk for finding heterogeneity (that is, significant variation in the results of different studies), thereby making analysis and interpretation of the results more difficult (27). If no heterogeneity is found even

when broad inclusion criteria are used, the results are more generalizable. Heterogeneity among studies can be useful, however, because it allows the researcher to study what caused it and generate new hypotheses (27, 28). Broad reviews can summarize large amounts of information in a single article; this may be more useful for readers but may require greater resources.

Although the inclusion criteria must be set before data collection begins, they should be flexible, provided that care is taken to avoid making changes that would be likely to introduce bias. Inclusion criteria should not be changed on the basis of the results of individual trials. It may, however, be reasonable to change the criteria if alternative, acceptable ways of defining the study population or intervention are discovered. Narrow criteria may also need to be broadened or broad criteria may need to be narrowed, depending on the amount of data found.

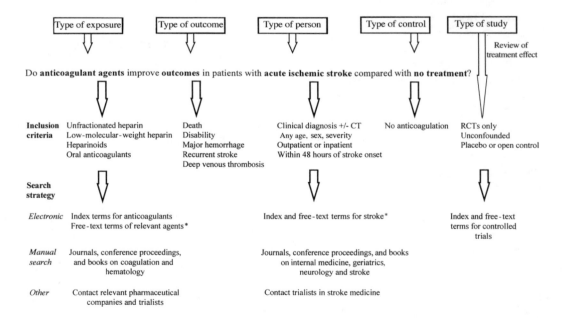

Figure 7.2 How a well-formulated question guides the review process. CT = computed tomography; RCT = randomized, controlled trial. * = see Appendix Table.

Locating Relevant Studies

As is the case with primary research studies, flaws in data collection can invalidate the results of a systematic review. As many relevant primary studies as possible (as resources allow) must be collected to minimize random error and bias. The first step is to decide which types of article must be retrieved with regard to the language of publication and publication status. For practical reasons, many systematic reviews restrict articles to the English language, but this practice is hard to justify. Existing evidence does not suggest that the quality of research varies by language of publication (29), and language restrictions can alter the results of systematic reviews by excluding available data (30). Some researchers (31) think that unpublished studies should be excluded because they have not been peer reviewed and therefore may have unreliable results. However, the most important influence on publication status is probably not scientific rigor but the nature of the results themselves. Publication bias—the selective publication of studies based on the direction and strength of their results (32)—affects all types of studies (including randomized, controlled trials [32-34]), but it seems to be a greater problem for small, nonrandomized studies (32, 33, 35). Because fewer studies with negative or null results are published than studies with larger, more positive results (32-34), reviews that exclude unpublished work are likely to overestimate the relation between the exposure and the outcome. As a consequence, treatment effects may be overestimated, making ineffective treatments seem effective (36, 37). Most researchers who do systematic reviews therefore think that unpublished studies should be included; if necessary, the results can be reanalyzed without the unpublished data (38).

Even among published studies, the nature of results varies according to the type of publication. Many primary studies are published as abstracts in conference proceedings, but only 50% of these go on to be published in full (39). Many studies that are published only as abstracts do not have statistically significant results; thus, excluding abstracts from systematic reviews may again limit the amount of data included in the review and introduce bias (39). Similar findings may apply to studies that were only published as letters or dissertations (40). Further data must be sought from the authors of letters and abstracts to determine whether they are eligible for inclusion in the review.

Search Strategies

Several complementary strategies can identify studies that are relevant to a systematic review (Table 7.3). Whichever methods are used, they must be reported in sufficient detail to allow replication. Again, a well-formulated question helps define the best search strategy (Figure 7.2).

The most commonly used strategy is searching electronic databases, such as MEDLINE or EMBASE. This method allows relatively quick access to large amounts of literature. Superficially, electronic searching seems simple: Enter a few appropriate terms, and the database should give back all the appropriate studies. In practice, however, electronic database searching is much more difficult. Studies have shown that depending on the topic, a MEDLINE search will identify only 32% to 91% of randomized, controlled trials published in jour-

Table 7.3   Sources of Relevant Studies

Electronic databases

Manual searching of journals, conference proceedings, and books

Reference lists

Existing study registries

Current-awareness publications

Pharmaceutical and appliance companies

Personal contact with colleagues and researchers

nals that are indexed by MEDLINE (41). This is in part due to inadequate indexing (attempts to improve the indexing of randomized, controlled trials are now under way [41, 42]) and in part to use of incorrect terms in the search strategy (41, 43). Reviewers must therefore take the time to plan their search systematically (43) and get help from persons who are experienced in using particular databases, such as medical librarians.

The first step in developing an electronic search is to include terms that refer to the disease or condition of interest (Appendix Table). Depending on the number of articles retrieved, the reviewer can restrict this search by combining it with searches for the exposure and study design of interest, then further restrict it to studies in humans. Because of the unreliability of indexing, the final search must include both controlled vocabulary terms, which vary with each database, and free text terms (41, 44). The best terms to use in the search can be determined by studying previously identified articles that meet the inclusion criteria. A provisional search can then be run on the most recent years and modified according to the articles found. Ideally, the performance of the electronic search should be validated by comparing its sensitivity against results obtained by doing a manual search of selected journals. For reviews that include randomized, controlled trials, an optimal MEDLINE search for randomized, controlled trials has been developed on behalf of the Cochrane Collaboration; a similar search should soon be available for EMBASE (45). As the number of terms in an electronic search increases, the number of both relevant and irrelevant articles identified increases. The reviewers must find the optimal balance between the two given available resources.

Even with an optimal search strategy, an electronic search will not identify articles in journals that are not indexed in the database (MEDLINE, for example, indexes about 4000 of 16 000 biomedical journals [41] and does not index issues before 1966); articles published in conference proceedings, because these are rarely indexed even if the proceedings are published in journals; unpublished articles; or articles published in books or dissertations. To minimize these problems, different databases can be searched to increase the coverage of journals; EMBASE, for example, indexes more than 1000 journals that are not found in MEDLINE. Many other general and subject-specific databases also exist, such as BIOSIS, CINAHL, PsychLit, and CancerLit. Other databases cover publications in languages other than English (46), conference proceedings (The International Scientific and Technical Proceedings database), dissertations (Index to UK Theses, Dissertation Abstracts), and unpublished literature (SIGLE [System for Information on the Grey Literature in Europe]) (41). However, these databases may be unavailable or costly to access, and each requires the development of a specific search strategy.

Given the problems of electronic searching, reviewers should use additional methods. A manual, page-by-page search of important journals and conference proceedings overcomes the problems of lack of coverage and poor indexing in databases. However, manual searching is very time- and labor-intensive, particularly if many journals must be searched (although volunteers can be trained to do this [47]). The Cochrane Collaboration is coordinating the manual searching of journals for randomized, controlled trials to minimize duplication of effort (45) and has also produced guidelines for quality control (48). Reference lists of studies and existing reviews are also useful sources of studies, but they do not identify a representative sample. Reference (citation) bias results in more favorable studies being cited more frequently (49). Reference tracking systems, such as the Science Citation Index, can also be used to identify the articles that quote important references. Many registries of studies already exist (45, 50) and should be searched. Current-awareness publications, such as *Current Contents*, are also useful to search because they include recently published research that has not yet been included in electronic databases.

Identifying unpublished studies is very difficult. Contacting companies can help identify industry-supported studies that involved particular drugs or appliances, but some companies may not be willing to share their data. Surveys of authors of previous research, experts in the field, and colleagues may also identify unpublished studies. However, these surveys are time-consuming and expensive and the retrieval rates can be very low. A survey of 42 000 obstetricians and pediatricians identified only 18 unpublished randomized, controlled trials in prenatal and obstetric care that had been completed more than 2 years previously (51). One solution to the problems of identifying unpublished studies would be to require registration of all research projects at their inception. Indeed, calls for such registration of clinical trials have repeatedly been made (32, 33, 41, 51-53), but major logistic and political hurdles must be overcome before this can become a reality (51, 53). In the meantime, researchers should be encouraged to submit their results for publication and to comply with requests for unpublished material because it is unethical not to do so (54).

The use of all the sources shown in Table 7.3 would create a comprehensive list of studies but would be costly in terms of time and money. Reviewers with limited resources must select the methods with the highest yield (55). Collaboration and avoidance of duplication are essential for decreasing the workload. These facts are recognized by such groups as the Cochrane Collaboration, which is coordinating an international effort to develop subject-specific registries of controlled clinical trials (45, 56). These registries are being combined (57) and, along with efforts to improve indexing of trials in MEDLINE (41, 42), may lead to the creation of a much-needed registry of all controlled clinical trials.

Conclusion

Considerable care is usually taken in the design and conduct of primary research studies. The same care should be taken in developing the protocol and the methods for a systematic review. The quality of a review largely depends on the time and attention spent at the outset on choosing an important question, formulating that question carefully, and planning the best ways to identify relevant primary data. For a researcher planning a systematic review, these investments will pay dividends later in terms of avoiding wasted time and effort and increasing the chance that the final review is scientifically, statistically, and clinically meaningful.

Key Points To Remember

- Choose an important, well-focused question.
- Refine the four major components of the question (people, exposure, control group, outcomes).
- Set clear, workable inclusion criteria.
- Take time to plan a sensible and thorough search strategy.
- Use multiple overlapping sources of data.
- Ensure that clinical and methodologic expertise and support are available.

Acknowledgments: The author thanks Cindy Mulrow, Andy Oxman, and Peter Sandercock for their helpful comments on this manuscript and thanks the clinical reviewer, Paul Speckart.

Grant Support: In part by a Wellcome Trust Research Training Fellowship in Clinical Epidemiology.

Appendix Table. Example of a MEDLINE Search for Studies of Anticoagulant Agents in Acute Ischemic Stroke[†]

Set	Search Term	Reports Found, *n*	Notes
1	CEREBRAL-INFARCTION/ all subheadings data	681	Searches in sets 1 through 4 used controlled vocabulary index terms (MeSH) in MEDLINE that covered acute ischemic stroke, starting with the most specific terms.
2	explode CEREBRAL-ISCHEMIA/all subheadings	1361	"Explode" means that the database searches for this term and other index terms subsumed under it.
3	explode CEREBRAL-EMBO-LISM-AND-THROMBOSIS/all subheadings	369	
4	CEREBROVASCULAR-DISORDERS/all subheadings	1359	
5	STROKE*	3041	Free-text searches for the word in the title and abstract of articles. The truncation term "*" means that any word beginning with "stroke" will be identified (for example, "stroke" and "strokes"). This search method is more sensitive and less specific.
6	1 or 2 or 3 or 4 or 5	4988	All searches for stroke articles were combined by using the Boolean "or" operator. This operator implies that an article only has to include any one of the terms to be retrieved.
7	explode ANTICOAGULANTS/ all subheadings	2398	Search for the intervention was done by using MeSH terms.
8	ANTICOAGUL*	1287	In sets 8 through 40, the titles and abstracts were searched for the intervention by using free-text terms for the many different anticoagulant agents. Use of truncation terms again improves sensitivity: for example, "Anticoagul*" identifies "anticoagulant" and "anticoagulation."
9	HEPARIN*	1950	
10	COUMARIN*	123	
11	DICUMAROL	10	
12	BISHYDROXYCOUMARIN	18	
13	ACENOCOUMAROL	32	
14	PHENPROCOUMON	24	
15	WARFARIN	318	
16	PHENINDIONE	7	
17	HIRUDIN	120	
18	ENOXAPARIN	36	In sets 18 through 20, the generic and trade names for the same drug were used. This highlights the need to use both in free-text searches.
19	PK 10169	1	
20	CLEXANE	1	
21	DALTEPARIN	2	In sets 21 through 23, the generic and trade names for the same drug were used.
22	KABI2165	0	
23	FRAGMIN	12	
24	NADROPARIN	15	In sets 24 through 27, the generic and trade names for the same drug were used.
25	CY 216	1	
26	FRAXIPARIN	6	
27	FRAXIPARINE	5	

Continued.

Appendix Table. Example of a MEDLINE Search for Studies of Anticoagulant Agents in Acute Ischemic Stroke[†]—*Continued.*

Set	Search Term	Reports Found, *n*	Notes
28	PARNAPARIN	2	
29	REVIPARIN	6	
30	TINZAPARIN	1	In sets 30 through 32, the generic and trade names for the same drug were used.
31	LOGIPARIN	6	
32	INNOHEP	0	
33	CY 222	1	
34	DANAPAROID	0	In sets 34 and 35, the generic and trade names for the same drug were used.
35	ORG 10172	10	
36	MESOGLYCAN	4	
37	DEXTRAN SULPHATE	22	Sets 37 and 38 highlight the need to use U.S. and British spellings.
38	DEXTRAN SULFATE	85	
39	HEPARIN	326	
40	PENTOSAN	24	
41	7 or 8 or 9 or 10 or 11 or 12 or 13 or 14 or 15 or 16 or 17 or 18 or 19 or 20 or 21 or 22 or 23 or 24 or 25 or 26 or 27 or 28 or 29 or 30 or 31 or 32 or 33 or 34 or 35 or 36 or 37 or 38 or 39 or 40	3946	Set 41 combines all the searches for the appropriate interventions by using the Boolean "or" operator. Including freetext terms added about 1500 references that were not found using the index term for anticoagulants.
42	6 and 41	285	Set 42 was the final search, combining the search for stroke-related articles with the search for anticoagulant-related articles by using the Boolean "and" operator. This operator implies that articles must include terms from both set 6 and set 41 to be retrieved. The search could be limited further if necessary by restricting it to human studies or by combining it with a search for a particular study design (such as randomized, controlled trials).[‡]

[†]Search was done in 1994 by using SilverPlatter, version 3.11.
[‡]See references 41 and 45.

References

1. **Chalmers I.** What do I want from health research and researchers when I am a patient? BMJ. 1995;310:1315-8.
2. **Goodare H, Smith R.** The rights of patients in research [Editorial]. BMJ. 1995;310:1277-8.
3. **Smith R.** What clinical information do doctors need? BMJ. 1996;313:1062-8.
4. **Eddy DM.** Selecting technologies for assessment. Int J Technol Assess Health Care. 1989;5:485-501.
5. **Lara ME, Goodman C, eds.** National Priorities for the Assessment of Clinical Conditions and Medical Technologies: Report of a Pilot Study. Council on Health Care Technology. Washington DC: National Academy Pr; 1990.
6. **Donaldson MS, Sox HC, eds.** Setting Priorities for Health Technology Assessment: A Model Process. Washington, DC: National Academy Pr; 1992.
7. **Standing Group on Health Technology.** 1994 Report. Department of Health, UK; 1994.
8. Evidence-based care: 1. Setting priorities: how important is this problem? Evidence-Based Care Resource Group. Can Med Assoc J. 1994;150:1249-54.
9. **Mumford CJ.** Beta interferon and multiple sclerosis: why the fuss? [Editorial] Q J Med. 1996:89:1-3.
10. **Antman EM, Lau J, Kupelnick B, Mosteller F, Chalmers TC.** A comparison of results of meta-analyses of randomized control trials and recommendations of clinical experts. Treatments for myocardial infarction. JAMA. 1992;268:240-8.
11. **Crowley P.** Corticosteroids prior to preterm delivery. In: Neilson JP, Crowther CA, Hodnett ED, Hofmeyr GJ, Keirse MJ, Renfrew MJ, eds. Pregnancy and Childbirth Module of The Cochrane Database of Systematic Reviews, updated 6 June 1996. Available in The Cochrane Library [on disk and CD-ROM]. The Cochrane Collaboration; Issue 2. Oxford: Update Software;

1996. Updated quarterly. Available from BMJ Publishing Group, London.

12. **Oxman AD, Cook DJ, Guyatt GH.** Users' guides to the medical literature. VI. How to use an overview. Evidence-Based Medicine Working Group. JAMA. 1994;272:1367-71.

13. **Eddy DM.** Clinical decision making: from theory to practice. Anatomy of a decision. JAMA. 1990;263:441-3.

14. **Fleming TR, DeMets DL.** Surrogate end points in clinical trials: are we being misled? Ann Intern Med. 1996;125:605-13.

15. **DeSilva RA, Hennekens CH, Lown B, Casscells W.** Lignocaine prophylaxis in acute myocardial infarction: an evaluation of randomised trials. Lancet. 1981;2:855-8.

16. **Drummond MF, Jefferson TO.** Guidelines for authors and peer reviewers of economic submissions to the BMJ. The BMJ Economic Evaluation Working Party. BMJ. 1996;313:275-83.

17. **Guyatt GH, Sackett DL, Cook DJ.** Users' guides to the medical literature. II. How to use an article about therapy or prevention. A. Are the results of the study valid? Evidence-Based Medicine Working Group. JAMA. 1993;270:2598-601.

18. **Schulz KF, Chalmers I, Hayes RJ, Altman DG.** Empirical evidence of bias. Dimensions of methodological quality associated with estimates of treatment effects in controlled trials. JAMA. 1995;273:408-12.

19. **Jaeschke R, Guyatt G, Sackett DL.** Users' guides to the medical literature. III. How to use an article about a diagnostic test. A. Are the results of the study valid? Evidence-Based Medicine Working Group. JAMA. 1994;271:389-91.

20. **Irwig L, Tosteson AN, Gatsonis C, Lau J, Colditz G, Chalmers TC, et al.** Guidelines for meta-analyses evaluating diagnostic tests. Ann Intern Med. 1994;120:667-76.

21. **Laupacis A, Wells G, Richardson WS, Tugwell P.** Users' guide to the medical literature. V. How to use an article about prognosis. Evidence-Based Medicine Working Group. JAMA. 1994;272:234-7.

22. **Willinger M, Hoffman HJ, Hartford RB.** Infant sleep position and risk for sudden death syndrome: report of meeting held January 13 and 14, 1994, National Institutes of Health, Bethseda, MD. Pediatrics. 1994;93:814-9.

23. **Counsell CE, Clarke MJ, Slattery J, Sandercock PA.** The miracle of DICE therapy for acute stroke: fact or fictional product of subgroup analysis? BMJ. 1994;309:1677-81.

24. **Peto R.** Why do we need systematic overviews of randomized trials? Stat Med. 1987;6:233-44.

25. **Yusuf S, Wittes J, Probstfield J, Tyroler HA.** Analysis and interpretation of treatment effects in subgroups of patients in randomized clinical trials. JAMA. 1991;266:93-8.

26. **Oxman AD, Guyatt GH.** A consumer's guide to subgroup analyses. Ann Intern Med. 1992;116:78-84.

27. **Dickersin K, Berlin JA.** Meta-analysis: state-of-the-science. Epidemiol Rev. 1992;14:154-76.

28. **Berlin JA.** Invited commentary: benefits of heterogeneity in meta-analyses of data from epidemiologic studies. Am J Epidemiol. 1995;142:383-7.

29. **Moher D, Fortin P, Jadad AR, J.ni P, Klassen T, Le Lorier J, et al.** Completeness of reporting of trials published in languages other than English: implications for conduct and reporting of systematic reviews. Lancet. 1996;347:363-6.

30. **Gregoire G, Derderian F, Le Lorier J.** Selecting the language of the publications included in a meta-analysis: is there a Tower of Babel bias? J Clin Epidemiol. 1995;48:159-63.

31. **Chalmers TC, Levin H, Sacks HS, Reitman D, Berrier J, Nagalingam R.** Meta-analysis of clinical trials as a scientific discipline. I: Control of bias and comparison with large co-operative trials. Stat Med. 1987;6:315-28.

32. **Dickersin K, Min YI.** Publication bias: the problem that won't go away. Ann N Y Acad Sci. 1993;703:135-46.

33. **Easterbrook PJ, Berlin JA, Gopalan R, Matthews DR.** Publication bias in clinical research. Lancet. 1991;337:867-72.

34. **Dickersin K, Chan S, Chalmers TC, Sacks HS, Smith H Jr.** Publication bias and clinical trials. Controlled Clin Trials. 1987;8:343-53.

35. **Newcombe RG.** Towards a reduction in publication bias. Br Med J (Clin Res Ed). 1987;295:656-9.

36. **Simes RJ.** Confronting publication bias: a cohort design for meta-analysis. Stat Med. 1987;6:11-29.

37. **Egger M, Smith GD.** Misleading meta-analysis. BMJ. 1995;310:752-4.

38. **Cook DJ, Guyatt GH, Ryan G, Clifton J, Buckingham L, Willan A, et al.** Should unpublished data be included in meta-analyses? Current convictions and controversies. JAMA. 1993;269:2749-53.

39. **Scherer RW, Dickersin K, Langenberg P.** Full publication of results initially presented in abstracts. A meta-analysis. JAMA. 1994;272:158-62.

40. **Glass GV, McGraw B, Smith ML.** Meta Analysis in Social Research. Beverly Hills, CA: Sage; 1981.

41. **Dickersin K, Scherer R, Lefebvre C.** Identifying studies for systematic reviews. BMJ. 1994;309:1286-91.

42. **Bero L, Rennie D.** The Cochrane Collaboration. Preparing, maintaining, and disseminating systematic reviews of the effects of health care. JAMA. 1995;274:1935-8.

43. **Jadad AR, McQuay HJ.** Searching the literature. Be systematic in your searching [Letter]. BMJ. 1993;307:66.

44. **Counsell CE, Fraser H.** Identifying relevant studies for systematic reviews [Letter]. BMJ. 1995;310:126.

45. **Dickersin K, Larsen K.** Section V: Establishing and maintaining an international register of RCTs. In: The Cochrane Collaboration Handbook. Available in The Cochrane Library [on disk and CD-ROM]. The Cochrane Collaboration; Issue 2. Oxford: Update Software; 1996. Available from BMJ Publishing Group, London.

46. **Tsutani K, Sakuma A.** How to access RCTs in Japan through network access from abroad. [Abstract]. In: Proceedings of the Second

International Cochrane Colloquium. Hamilton, Ontario, Canada, 1-4 October 1994.

47. How good are volunteers at searching for published randomized controlled trials? The OSTR Collaborative Group. Ottawa Stroke Trials Registry. Fundam Clin Pharmacol. 1995;9:384-6.

48. Journal Hand Search Manual. Baltimore: Cochrane Center; 1995.

49. **Gotzsche P.** Reference bias in reports of drug trials. Br Med J (Clin Res Ed). 1987;295:654-6.

50. **Easterbrook PJ.** Directory of registries of clinical trials. Stat Med. 1992;11:345-423.

51. **Hetherington J, Dickersin K, Chalmers I, Meinert CL.** Retrospective and prospective identification of unpublishedcontrolled trials: lessons from a survey of obstetricians and pediatricians. Pediatrics. 1989;84:374-80.

52. **Simes RJ.** Publication bias: the case for an international registry of clinical trials. J Clin Oncol. 1986;4:1529-41.

53. Making clinical trialists register. Lancet. 1991;338:244-5.

54. **Chalmers I.** Underreporting research is scientific misconduct. JAMA. 1990;263:1405-8.

55. **Jadad AR, McQuay HJ.** A high-yield strategy to identify randomized controlled trials for systematic reviews. Online J Curr Clin Trials. 1993;Doc No 33:3973 words, 39 paragraphs.

56. **Sackett D.** Section I. The Cochrane Collaboration. In: The Cochrane Collaboration Handbook. Available in The Cochrane Library [on disk and CD-ROM]. The Cochrane Collaboration; Issue 2. Oxford: Update Software; 1996. Updated quarterly. Available from BMJ Publishing Group, London.

57. The Cochrane Controlled Trials Register. Availablein The Cochrane Library [database on disk and CD-ROM]. The Cochrane Collaboration; Issue 2. Oxford: Update Software; 1996. Updated quarterly. Available from BMJ Publishing Group, London.

Chapter 8

Selecting and Appraising Studies for a Systematic Review

Maureen O. Meade, MD, FRCPC, MSc; and W. Scott Richardson, MD

After thoroughly searching the potentially relevant literature for a systematic review, reviewers face the sequential tasks of selecting studies for inclusion and appraising these studies. Methodical, impartial, and reliable strategies are necessary for these two tasks because systematic reviews are retrospective exercises and are therefore prone to both bias and random error. To plan for study selection, reviewers begin with a focused clinical question and choose selection criteria that reflect this question. A detailed selection protocol that specifies the study designs and publication status of articles to be included is often helpful. Selection criteria are itemized on customized forms and are used to examine each potentially relevant primary study, usually by two different reviewers. In planning the critical appraisal of included studies, reviewers decide which clinical and methodologic study features require documentation. After choosing methods for evaluating study quality, reviewers construct customized appraisal forms and an explicit protocol for the actual evaluation. Some of the techniques commonly used to minimize the potential for error in study appraisal include duplicate, independent examination; blinding to study results and other identifying features of each article; and correspondence with study authors to clarify issues.

Ultimately, primary studies should be selected, appraised, and reported in sufficient detail to allow readers to judge the applicability of the review to clinical practice and to clarify the strength of the inferences that can be drawn from the review.

This chapter outlines methods with which to search the literature for studies on the clinical question that generates a systematic review (1). Herein, we discuss the subsequent steps of selecting and appraising studies for a review. Both of these steps involve important judgments that can influence the results of a review. In selecting studies, reviewers judge the relevance of the studies to the review question. In appraising studies, reviewers judge numerous features of design and analysis. Some of these judgments are easy to make; others are more difficult and prone to error.

To be confident in their decisions, reviewers should use methods that are reliable (the results do not change if the procedure is repeated), impartial (not influenced by the study results), and explicit (unambiguous) (2). These strategies for selection and appraisal are sensible, and they distinguish most systematic reviews from most narrative reviews. However, evidence to support the importance of some of the methods we suggest is either scant or conflicting; readers are referred to the original research on these approaches for more details.

Selecting Studies for Systematic Reviews

If reviewers perform a comprehensive search of the literature using the methods described in Chapter 7 (1), they will probably have assembled a large sample of articles. This sample will include most (ideally, all) studies that are relevant to the review question (that is, the sensitivity of the search will be high). Inevitably, because such a wide net is cast, articles not pertinent to the clinical question will be retrieved (that is, the specificity of the search will be modest). Thus, the reviewers' next task is to sort through all of the potentially relevant articles and select those that will be included in the review. To do so, reviewers adopt several of the tactics listed in Tables 8.1 and 8.2 for planning and executing the selection process (in effect, improving the specificity of the search); these tactics are described below.

Begin with a Well-Built Clinical Question

Reviewers should ensure that the question for review includes the elements of a well-built clinical question (3, 4): the

Table 8.1   Planning Study Selection

Begin with a well-built clinical question
Choose selection criteria that fit the clinical question
Specify the types of study design to be included
Specify criteria related to type and form of publication
Construct and pretest selection forms
Write a detailed protocol

patients of interest, the main interventions under investigation, the comparison interventions, and the clinical outcomes of interest. By including these elements, reviewers can better focus the selection process.

Choose Selection Criteria That Fit the Clinical Question

Consider a systematic review of the effectiveness of a drug treatment (for example, a proton-pump inhibitor) for patients with a particular disorder (such as esophageal reflux). Reviewers need to decide whether to include studies of patients with any symptoms of reflux, only those with "classic" symptoms, or only those in whom definitive diagnostic tests have confirmed the presence of reflux. In addition, reviewers might choose to include studies of patients with different comorbid conditions; patients from different demographic or geographic or cultural backgrounds; or patients from different health systems, such as inpatient or community populations.

Similarly, reviewers should use selection criteria that reflect the main and comparison interventions of interest. In our esophageal reflux example, reviewers would need to decide whether to include studies of a particular drug or studies of all agents in that drug's class and whether to include studies of any dose and regimen or only studies with a specific regimen. For the comparison interventions, the reviewers would decide whether to include studies that compare the experimental drug with

Table 8.2   Strategies for Selecting and Appraising
Studies

Follow the protocol and record your prognosis

Have two or more investigators review each study
   independently

Consider "blinding" to study results

Correspond with authors to confirm study
   characteristics

alternate treatments (such as antacids or histamine-2-receptor antagonists), with placebo, or with both.

For the clinical outcomes, reviewers have analogous tasks of defining the outcomes and translating them into criteria. In our example, the reviewers would start by listing each clinical outcome (for example, whether the outcome was endoscopic or clinical and whether it focused on cure or persistence) and then decide whether to include studies that reported any outcome or only those with certain clinically important outcomes (such as improvement in symptoms at 1 year).

After thoroughly considering each element of the review question, reviewers compile a set of explicit selection criteria. When these criteria are not explicit, the results of the review are more prone to error (5, 6). Reporting the selection criteria used in a review is extremely important to readers because the criteria indicate the relevance of the review to the readers' clinical practice.

Specify the Types of Study Design To Be Included

After creating selection criteria that appropriately reflect the review question, reviewers should consider which study designs to include. Ideally, reviewers choose study designs that are most likely to produce valid results. For example, to answer questions about therapy or harm, reviewers may want to include randomized trials (7) because they provide more accurate estimates of benefit or harm than do

cohort studies, case-control studies, and case series (8). In reality, however, randomized trials may not be conducted to address questions of harm (9). Therefore, reviewers need to consider which study designs are likely to be available to answer their question; this information may necessitate modification of originally conceptualized selection criteria to incorporate observational (nonexperimental) studies.

Specify Criteria Related to Type and Form of Publication

Reviewers also need to consider issues related to type and form of publication. Ideally, all of the relevant studies would be published as peer-reviewed journal articles. However, some completed studies may be published only as abstracts, in non-peer-reviewed form, or not at all. Reviewers decide whether to include these incompletely reported studies when planning their literature search. By including all articles in various stages of publication and subjecting them to rigorous critical appraisal, reviewers minimize the threat of publication bias (the preferential reporting of studies with positive results) (10-12), which could generate misleading reviews. Other studies may be reported more than once. To avoid over-representing duplicate studies in the review, investigators should plan to look for and exclude duplicate publications (13). Finally, because studies may be published in different languages and because excluding studies published in different languages may bias the results of reviews (14, 15), articles should be included, as appropriate, regardless of the language of publication (translating as necessary). Limited time and resources, however, may preclude such an approach.

Construct and Pretest Selection Forms

After deciding on selection criteria, reviewers can prepare customized forms that contain checklists of the selection criteria (Figure 8.1). Using these forms can simplify the selection process, increase reliability, and provide a record of the judgments made about each study. After drafting form prototypes, reviewers "pretest" these forms for clarity, ease of application, and reliability. To pretest the forms, two or more independent reviewers typically apply them to a random sample of studies identified by the literature search. Reviewers compare their results to identify sources of ambiguity and then revise the forms accordingly. If the revisions are substantial, this process may need to be repeated before the forms can be used.

Write a Detailed Protocol

Having a selection protocol as part of a larger protocol for the entire review helps reviewers in two ways. First, it provides a document that explicitly states the review question and the selection criteria, making the process accountable. Reviewers can later return to the protocol for guidance in resolving disagreements about article selection. Second, the selection protocol identifies what work will be done, by whom, in what manner, when, and for what reason; thus, it provides a mode of communication within the review team.

When reviewers have a very large sample of studies from which to select, they can simplify this task by reviewing all of the titles, then the abstracts, and then the full articles, excluding studies that do not meet one or more selection criteria at each step. In doing so, reviewers should record (on the selection forms) the reasons for exclusion. After reviewers have selected studies for the systematic review, they will move to

---

Citation:_____

Level of Review (please check):   Title __   Abstract __   Article __

Name of Reviewer:_____   Date of Review:_____

Selection Criteria

(Please indicate with a check mark if each of the following criteria are met.)

Population	Did study patients have documented esophageal or gastric varices?
	Did study patients previously have an episode of variceal bleeding?
Study Intervention	Did at least one study group receive oral β-blockers?
Control Intervention	Did one study group receive no prophylactic therapy?
Outcomes	Was one of the measured outcomes a documented episode of variceal bleeding?
ACTION:	Include __ Exclude __

Please list reason(s) for exclusion: _____

_____

Figure 8.1 Example of a form that might be developed for the selection of studies for a systematic review evaluating the efficacy of β-blockers for secondary prevention of variceal bleeding.

the next task of critical appraisal. This procedure also requires careful planning.

Appraising Studies for Systematic Reviews

Reviewers appraise the studies selected for review with three objectives in mind: 1) to understand the validity of the studies, 2) to uncover reasons for differences among study results other than chance, and 3) to provide readers with sufficient information with which to judge for themselves the applicability of the systematic review to their clinical practice. To achieve these goals, reviewers use the strategies outlined in Tables 8.2 and 8.3 to carefully reexamine many important features of the primary studies.

Examine Important Clinical Features

Although the selection criteria for a systematic review define the population, interventions, and outcomes of interest, the appraisal process involves a detailed assessment of the patients (for example, high, medium, or low risk), the study interventions (for example, frequency, degree, and duration), and the outcome measurements (for example, definitions and degree of surveillance) in each study. Variations among any of these design features may be an important source of variation among study results. Appraisals of primary studies that reveal differences among study protocols may direct subsequent subgroup analyses if the results are statistically combined.

Consider, for example, a systematic review of the accuracy of persantine thallium scanning in predicting postoperative myocardial infarction in patients who undergo noncardiac vascular repair. Because the accuracy of the test may vary among patients with different degrees of risk (16), reviewers should document risk factors for myocardial infarction (for example, age; diabetes; hypertension; and history of congestive heart failure, unstable angina, or myocardial infarction) for the patients in each study. Similarly, reviewers should record the methods used to administer the test, including intravenous compared with oral administration of persantine, planar compared with single-photon emission computed tomography, and the time interval for delayed images. Finally, reviewers should record details related to outcome measurement, including precise definitions of myocardial infarction and the completeness and duration of follow-up.

Examine the Quality of Study Methods

The research methods used in the primary studies reflect the "quality" of the studies. In this sense, quality refers to the extent to which the study design, conduct, and analysis minimize the potential for bias. Biased primary studies are obviously more likely to provide misleading results and, by extension, will generate misleading systematic reviews. Therefore, reviewers should critically appraise the methods of all primary studies. High-quality studies use methods that are most likely to provide a true estimate of the benefit or harm of a treatment or exposure, the diagnostic accuracy of a test, or a particular prognosis. Current standards for evaluating the quality of studies on therapy, prevention, diagnosis, prognosis, and harm (4) are the basis of quality assessments in systematic reviews (Table 8.4).

Three methodologic features have been empirically shown to influence the results of studies about therapy: randomization, concealment of randomization, and blinding (7, 17-19). Random allocation to treatment means that investigators ensure that each patient entering the trial has an equal chance of getting into each treatment

Table 8.3   Planning Study Appraisal

Examine important clinical features

Evaluate the quality of study methods

Construct and pretest appraisal forms

Write a detailed protocol

Table 8.4   Abridged Checklist for Evaluating the Quality of Study Methods for Various Study Designs*

Therapy	Were patients randomly assigned to treatment?
	Was follow-up sufficiently thorough and were all of the patients accounted for?
	Were patients analyzed according to the groups to which they were randomly assigned?
Diagnosis	Was there an independent, blinded comparison with a reference (gold) standard?
	Did the patient sample include an appropriate spectrum of patients to whom the diagnostic test will be applied in clinical practice?
Harm	Were comparison groups clearly identified that were similar with respect to important determinants of outcome (other than the one of interest)?
	Were outcomes and exposures measured in the same way in the groups being compared?
Prognosis	Was there a representative patient sample at a well-defined point in the course of disease?
	Was follow-up sufficiently thorough?

*Adapted from Oxman and colleagues (4) with permission.

group. Concealment means that investigators are unaware of the treatment group to which a patient will be randomly assigned before the patient enters the trial. Conversely, blinding refers to the masking of caregivers, patients, and research personnel to treatment allocation after a patient has been entered into a trial. Nonrandomized studies (17, 18), unconcealed randomization (18, 19), and unblinded studies (7) all tend to overestimate the effectiveness of therapeutic interventions. A summary of anonymous reports from investigators describes the extreme measures that have been used to unconceal treatment group allocation (20). Therefore, in randomized trials, the methods of randomization should be clearly documented so that readers and reviewers can evaluate this important methodologic feature. Unfortu-

nately, the randomization process is inadequately described in most published reports (19, 21, 22).

Reviewers may choose from among many techniques for assessing the methodologic quality of included studies. First, the simplest approach is to use a few components that itemize the key design features (Table 8.4). Second, reviewers may develop more comprehensive checklists. Although they are generally more complex, customized checklists are particularly helpful for documenting the quality of studies of diagnostic tests or prognosis. Third, reviewers may use quantitative scales that provide a summary score for the overall quality of individual studies. A recent review identified nine checklists and 25 different scales for assessing the quality of primary studies for systematic reviews, although only one checklist was rigorously developed (23). Most quality assessment scales that have been published for general use do not include items that are known to influence the ability of the study to provide a true (unbiased) estimate of treatment effect. For example, one published scale includes an item related to the reporting of sample size calculation (24). Neglecting to report the sample size calculation may reflect the omission of an a priori sample size determination or could reflect poor reporting or editing; however, these oversights do not result in a biased estimate of efficacy. When systematic reviews use scales for measuring methodologic quality, points are allotted for methodologic features that minimize bias (such as randomization and blinding) (Table 8.4). These points are summed to provide a numerical descriptor of overall quality: the methodologic quality score.

Methodologic quality scores can be applied in many ways in systematic reviews (25). For example, they may be used to evaluate the influence of quality on study results. One method is to graphically plot study results against methodologic quality scores to evaluate any association. This practice may be useful if the methods of individual studies vary widely. In addition, methodologic quality scores can guide qualitative and quantitative analyses. For example, reviewers may choose a cutoff score to select studies for pooling in secondary analyses. Ideally, the cutoff score should be chosen a priori on the basis of biological rationale rather than on the basis of study results. Similarly, quality scores may be used to perform "sensitivity" analyses, in which subsamples of selected studies featuring specific design characteristics or threshold quality scores are statistically combined. Finally, reviewers may use these scores to perform weighted analyses, in which the relative weight of an individual study in a meta-analysis is determined by the magnitude of the methodologic quality score. The application of methodologic quality scores in systematic reviews must be considered in light of the scores' limitations. For instance, assigning relative values to specific study methods to generate a quality score is largely an arbitrary and unscientific process. Furthermore, the assumption of a direct and universal relation between study quality and results may be unfounded. When one group of investigators applied a particular quality scale to studies reviewed in seven meta-analyses published in the 1980s, no association between quality scores and study results was shown (26). These techniques of data analysis will be discussed in detail in the next chapter of this book (27).

Construct and Pretest Appraisal Forms

Just as reviewers are well advised to construct standardized forms for the selection process, they should develop and test forms for appraising the studies selected for review. Consultation with clinical experts or methodologists help verify that the forms include a comprehensive list of important study features particular to the study design and clinical topic.

Write a Detailed Protocol

Just as reviewers find it useful to create a protocol for the selection process, they should develop an explicit protocol outlining the appraisal procedures.

Strategies for Executing Study Selection and Appraisal

Follow the Protocol and Record Progress

After writing protocols for study selection and appraisal that are based on sound criteria and use well-built forms, reviewers are well prepared to follow the protocol and record their progress. As each article is reviewed, selection and appraisal forms will provide a record of the judgments made about each study. This information can be invaluable when reviewers prepare a log of excluded studies for publication or a table that summarizes the methodologic quality of included studies.

Review Each Study Independently and in Duplicate

Even when following explicit criteria for selecting and appraising studies, reviewers can face difficult decisions. To minimize the potential for error in these judgments, we recommend that two or more investigators review each study independently. Reviewers often measure their inter-rater agreement across studies for each item on the selection and appraisal forms using a κ statistic (which measures agreement beyond the play of chance) (28, 29). Although agreement between two reviewers does not guarantee accurate decisions, the higher the agreement among reviewers, the more confidence readers can have in the results of the review (30). When reviewers disagree, the reasons for these disagreements should be explored. Often, reviewers can quickly clarify the source of the disagreement if they both refer to the article and the review protocol. An alternative is to enlist other collaborators in resolving disagreements, as specified in the protocol. Resolving disagreements by enlightened discussion is often preferred to voting by majority because the majority might be incorrect. For future reference, reviewers should record these disagreements and how they are resolved.

Consider "Blinding" to Study Results

Investigators can consider blinding reviewers to study results in order to make their judgments as impartial as possible. This task may be as simple as providing reviewers with just the Methods sections from the articles being considered. Unfortunately, relevant information is often dispersed throughout the Results and Discussion sections; therefore, a great deal of cutting and pasting may be required. Furthermore, if a reviewer recognizes the authors, their institutions, or the date or journal of publication, he or she may be influenced by prior knowledge of the study or its results. Electrically scanning journal pages and printing them after relevant identifiers have been eliminated are a modern approach to blinding in this context; however, this process can be extremely labor-intensive and requires a high level of judgment.

One study showed that blinded quality assessment of primary studies produces significantly lower and more consistent scores than do open assessments (31). However, a recent randomized trial evaluated study selection and data abstraction either by assessment that was blinded to author, institution, and journal or by open assessment. Blinding had neither a clinically nor a statistically significant effect on the summary odds ratio of these five meta-analyses (32). Although blinding reviewers to study results and all identifying characteristics continues to be advocated in some circles, the theoretical benefits of these efforts must be weighed against the effort involved in blinding.

Correspond with Authors To Confirm Study Characteristics

Some articles may contain incomplete or confusing descriptions of the study methods, leading to incorrect selection decisions or critical appraisal. To overcome this problem, reviewers can ask for collaboration from the authors for clarification. Such correspondence and subsequent decisions of the review team should also be recorded for future reference.

Conclusions

The selection and appraisal of studies for a systematic review should use methodical, reliable, and impartial methods. Familiarity with the principles of critical appraisal is fundamental to these steps. Highlighting the differences in study methods through critical appraisal facilitates an evaluation of the inconsistencies among study results. Furthermore, the appraisal exercises help to establish the strength of inferences that can be drawn from the review. This exercise may also guide further research on the topic.

After applying the strategies presented in this chapter to the fruits of a literature search, systematic reviewers are prepared to move on to the qualitative and quantitative synthesis of study results. The strategies for combining studies for systematic reviews, including statistical analyses, will be presented in the next chapter of this book (27).

Key Points To Remember

- In selecting studies for review, investigators must judge the degree of each study's relevance to the clinical question and critically assess study design features.
- To be confident in their decisions, reviewers need to use methods of study selection and appraisal that are reliable, impartial, and explicit.
- When selecting from a large sample of studies, reviewers can simplify the task

by first reviewing all of the titles, then the abstracts, and then the full articles, excluding studies at each step that do not meet one or more selection criteria.

• By including all types of documents (for example, peer-reviewed publications, abstracts, unpublished reports) and subjecting them equally to rigorous critical appraisal, reviewers minimize the possibility of publication bias.

• Reviewers must appraise the studies selected for a systematic review with three objectives in mind: to understand the rigor of the studies to be included, to uncover reasons for differences among study results, and to provide readers with sufficient information with which to judge the applicability of the review to their clinical practice.

• Three methodologic features have been empirically shown to influence the results of studies about therapy: randomization, concealment of randomization, and blinding.

Acknowledgment: The authors thank the clinical reviewer, Norman J. Wilder.

References

1. **Counsell C.** Formulating the questions and locating primary studies for inclusion in systematic reviews. Ann Intern Med. 1997;127:380-7.
2. **Oxman AD, ed.** Section VI: Preparing and Maintaining Systematic Reviews: The Cochrane Collaboration Handbook. Oxford: Cochrane Collaboration; 1994:28-40.
3. **Richardson WS, Wilson MC, Nishikawa J, Hayward RS.** The well-built clinical question: a key to evidence-based decisions [Editorial]. ACP J Club. 1995;123:A12-3.
4. **Oxman AD, Sackett DL, Guyatt GH.** Users' guides to the medical literature. I. How to get started. The Evidence-Based Medicine Working Group. JAMA. 1993;270:2093-5.
5. **Chalmers TC, Levin H, Sacks HS, Reitman D, Berrier J, Nagalingam R.** Meta-analysis of clinical trials as a scientific discipline. I: Control of bias and comparison with large co-operative trials. Stat Med. 1987;6:315-25.
6. **Chalmers TC, Berrier J, Sacks HS, Levin H, Reitman D, Nagalingam R.** Meta-analysis of clinical trials as a scientific discipline. II: Replicate variability and comparison of studies that agree and disagree. Stat Med. 1987;6:733-44.
7. **Schulz K, Chalmers I, Hayes RJ, Altman DG.** Empirical evidence of bias. Dimensions of methodological quality associated with estimates of treatment effects in controlled clinical trials. JAMA. 1995;273:408-12.
8. **Cook DJ, Guyatt GH, Laupacis A, Sackett DL, Goldberg RJ.** Clinical recommendations using levels of evidence for antithrombotic agents. Chest. 1995;108(4 Suppl):227S-30S.
9. **Levine M, Walter S, Lee H, Haines T, Holbrook A, Moyer V.** Users' guides to the medical literature IV. How to use an article about harm. The Evidence-Based Medicine Working Group. JAMA. 1994;271:1615-9.
10. **Easterbrook PJ, Berlin JA, Gopalan R, Mathews DR.** Publication bias in clinical research. Lancet. 1991;337:867-72.
11. **Cook DJ, Guyatt GH, Ryan G, Clifton J, Buckingham L, Willan A, et al.** Should unpublished data be included in meta-analyses? Current convictions and controversies. JAMA. 1993;269:2749-53.
12. **Scherer RW, Dickersin K, Langenberg P.** Full publication of results initially presented in abstracts. A meta-analysis. JAMA. 1994;272:158-62.
13. **Gotzsche P.** Multiple publications of reports of drug trials. Eur J Clin Pharmacol. 1989;36:429-32.
14. **Gregoire G, Derderian F, Le Lorier J.** Selecting the language of the publications included in a meta-analysis: is there a Tower of Babel bias? J Clin Epidemiol. 1995;48:159-63.
15. **Egger M, Zellweger-Zahner T, Schneider M, Junker C, Lengeler C, Antes G.** Language bias in randomised controlled trials published in English and German. Lancet. 1997;350:326-9.
16. **Ransohoff DF, Feinstein AR.** Problems of spectrum and bias in evaluating the efficacy of diagnostic tests. N Engl J Med. 1978;299:926-30.
17. **Sacks HS, Chalmers TC, Smith H Jr.** Randomized versus historical assignment in controlled clinical trials. N Engl J Med. 1983;309:1353-7.
18. **Chalmers TC, Celano P, Sacks HS, Smith H Jr.** Bias in treatment assignment in controlled clinical trials. N Engl J Med. 1983;309:1358-61.
19. **Schulz KF, Chalmers I, Grimes DA, Altman DG.** Assessing the quality of randomization from reports of controlled trials published in obstetrics and gynecology journals. JAMA. 1994;272:125-8.
20. **Schulz KF.** Subverting randomization in clinical trials. JAMA. 1995; 274: 1456-8.
21. **Altman DG, Dore CJ.** Randomization and baseline comparisons in clinical trials. Lancet. 1990;335:149-53.
22. **Williams DH, Davis CE.** Reporting of assignment methods in clinical trials. Control Clin Trials. 1994;15:294-8.
23. **Moher D, Jadad AR, Nichol G, Penman M, Tugwell P, Walsh S.** Assessing the quality of randomized controlled trials: an annotated bibliography of scales and checklists. Control Clin Trials. 1995;16:62-73.
24. **Chalmers TC, Smith H, Blackburn B, Silverman B, Schroeder B, Reitman D, et al.** A

method for assessing the quality of a randomized control trial. Control Clin Trials. 1981;2:31-49.

25. **Detsky AS, Naylor CD, O'Rourke K, McGeer AJ, L'Abbe KA.** Incorporating variations in the quality of individual randomized trials into meta-analysis. J Clin Epidemiol. 1992;45:255-65.

26. **Emerson JD, Burdick E, Hoaglin DC, Mosteller F, Chalmers TC.** An empirical study of the possible relation of treatment differences to quality scores in controlled randomized clinical trials. Control Clin Trials. 1990;11:339-52.

27. **Lau J.** Combining data quantitatively in systematic reviews. Ann Intern Med. 1997;127:820-26.

28. **Streiner DL, Norman GR.** Reliability. In: Health Measurement Scales: A Practical Guide to Their Development and Use. 2d ed. Oxford: Oxford Univ Pr; 1995.

29. **Altman DG.** Measuring agreement. In: Practical Statistics for Medical Research. London: Chapman and Hall; 1991.

30. **Oxman AD, Cook DJ, Guyatt GH.** Users' guides to the medical literature. VI. How to use an overview. The Evidence-Based Medicine Working Group. JAMA. 1994;272:1367-71.

31. **Jadad AR, Moore RA, Carrol D, Jenkinson C, Reynolds DJ, Gavaghan DJ, et al.** Assessing the quality of randomized clinical trials: is blinding necessary? Control Clin Trials. 1996;17:1-12.

32. **Berlin JA, Miles CG, Crigliano MD, Conill AM, Goldmann DR, Horowitz DA, et al.** Does blinding of readers affect the results of meta-analyses? Results of a randomized trial. Online J Curr Clin Trials. Document no. 205.

Chapter 9

Quantitative Synthesis in Systematic Reviews

Joseph Lau, MD; John P.A. Ioannidis, MD; and Christopher H. Schmid, PhD

The final common pathway for most systematic reviews is a statistical summary of the data, or meta-analysis. The complex methods used in meta-analyses should always be complemented by clinical acumen and common sense in designing the protocol of a systematic review, deciding which data can be combined, and determining whether data should be combined. Both continuous and binary data can be pooled. Most meta-analyses summarize data from randomized trials, but other applications, such as the evaluation of diagnostic test performance and observational studies, have also been developed. The statistical methods of meta-analysis aim at evaluating the diversity (heterogeneity) among the results of different studies, exploring and explaining observed heterogeneity, and estimating a common pooled effect with increased precision. Fixed-effects models assume that an intervention has a single true effect, whereas random-effects models assume that an effect may vary across studies. Meta-regression analyses, by using each study rather than each patient as a unit of observation, can help to evaluate the effect of individual variables on the magnitude of an observed effect and thus may sometimes explain why study results differ. It is also important to assess the robustness of conclusions through sensitivity analyses and a formal evaluation of potential sources of bias, including publication bias and the effect of the quality of the studies on the observed effect.

A quantitative systematic review, or meta-analysis, uses statistical methods to combine the results of multiple studies. Meta-analyses have been done for systematic reviews of therapeutic trials, diagnostic test evaluations, and epidemiologic studies.

Although the statistical methods involved may at first appear to be mathematically complex, their purpose is simple. They are trying to answer four basic questions. Are the results of the different studies similar? To the extent that they are similar, what is the best overall estimate? How precise and robust is this estimate? Finally, can dissimilarities be explained? This chapter provides some guidance in understanding the key technical aspects of the quantitative approach to these questions. We have avoided using equations and statistical notations; interested readers will find implementations of the described methods in the listed references. We focus here on the quantitative synthesis of reports of randomized, controlled, therapeutic trials because far more meta-analyses on therapeutic studies than on other types of studies have been published.

For practical reasons, we present a stepwise description of the tasks that are performed when statistical methods are used to combine data. These tasks are 1) deciding whether to combine data and defining what to combine, 2) evaluating the statistical heterogeneity of the data, 3) estimating a common effect, 4) exploring and explaining heterogeneity, 5) assessing the potential for bias, and 6) presenting the results.

Deciding Whether To Combine Data and Defining What To Combine

By the time one performs a quantitative synthesis, certain decisions should already have been made about the formulation of the question and the selection of included studies. These topics were discussed in Chapters 7 and 8 (previously published as articles in the *Annals* series on systematic reviews [1,2]). Statistical tests cannot compensate for lack of common sense, clinical acumen, and biological plausibility in the design of the protocol of a meta-analysis. Thus, a reader of a systematic review should always address these issues before evaluating the statistical methods that have been used and the results that have been generated. Combining poor-quality data, overly biased data, or data that do not make sense can easily produce unreliable results.

The data to be combined in a meta-analysis are usually either binary or continuous. Binary data involve a yes/no categorization (for example, death or survival). Continuous data take a range of values (for example, change in diastolic blood pressure after antihypertensive treatment, measured in mm Hg).

When one is comparing groups of patients, binary data can be summarized by using several measures of treatment effect that were discussed in Chapter 3, (previously published in the Annals series [3]). These measures include the risk ratio, the odds ratio, the risk difference, and, when study duration is important, the incidence rate. Another useful clinical measure, the number needed to treat (NNT), is derived from the inverse of the risk difference (3). Treatment effect measures, such as the risk ratio and the odds ratio, provide an estimate of the relative efficacy of an intervention, whereas the risk difference describes the intervention's absolute benefit. The various measures of treatment effect offer complementary information, and all should be examined (4).

Continuous data can be summarized by the raw mean difference between the treatment and control groups when the treatment effect is measured on the same scale (for example, diastolic blood pressure in mm Hg), by the standardized mean difference when different scales are used to measure the same treatment effect (for example, different pain scales being combined), or by the correlation coefficients between two continuous variables (5). The standardized mean difference, also called the effect size, is obtained by dividing the difference between the mean in the treatment group and the mean in the control group by the SD in the control group.

Evaluating the Statistical Heterogeneity of the Data

This step is intended to determine whether the results of the different studies are similar (homogeneous). It is important to determine this question before combining any data. To do so, one must calculate the magnitude of the statistical diversity (heterogeneity) of the treatment effect that exists among the different sets of data.

Statistical diversity can be thought of as attributable to one or both of two causes. First, study results can differ because of random sampling error. Even if the true effect is the same in each study, the results of different studies would be expected to vary randomly around the true common *fixed* effect. This diversity is called the within-study variance. Second, each study may have been drawn from a different population, depending on the particular patients chosen and the interventions and conditions unique to the study. Therefore, even if each study enrolled a large patient sample, the treatment effect would be expected to differ. These differences, called *random* effects, describe the between-study variation with regard to an overall mean of the effects of all of the studies that could be undertaken.

The test most commonly used to assess the statistical significance of between-study heterogeneity is based on the chi-square distribution (6). It provides a measure of the sum of the squared differences between the results observed and the results expected in each study, under the assumption that each study estimates the same common treatment effect. A large total deviation indicates that a single common treatment effect is unlikely. Any pooled estimate calculated must account for the between-study heterogeneity. In practice, this test has low sensitivity for detecting heterogeneity, and it has been suggested that a liberal significance level, such as 0.1, should be used (6).

Estimating a Common Effect

The questions that this step tries to answer are 1) To the extent that data are similar, what is their best common point estimate of a therapeutic effect, and 2) how precise is this estimate? The mathematical process involved in this step generally involves combining (pooling) the results of different studies into an overall estimate. Compared with the results of individual studies, pooled results can increase statistical power and lead to more precise estimates of treatment effect.

Each study is given a weight according to the precision of its results. The rationale is that studies with narrow CIs should be weighted more heavily than studies with greater uncertainty. The precision is generally expressed by the inverse of the variance of the estimate of each study. The variance has two components: the variance of the individual study and the variance between different studies. When the between-study variance is found to be or assumed to be zero, each study is simply weighted by the inverse of its own variance, which is a function of the study size and the number of events in the study. This approach characterizes a fixed-effects model, as exemplified by the Mantel-Haenszel method (7, 8) or the Peto method (9) for dichotomous data. The Peto method has been particularly popular in the past. It has the advantage of simple calculation; however, although it is appropriate in most cases, it may introduce large biases if the data are unbalanced (10, 11). On the other hand, random-effects models also add the between-study variance to the within-study variance of each individual study when the pooled mean of the random effects is calculated. The random-effects model most commonly used for dichotomous data is the DerSimonian and Laird estimate of the between-study variance (12). Fixed- and random-effects models for continuous data have also been described (13). Pooled results are generally reported as a point estimate and CI, typically a 95% CI.

Other quantitative techniques for combining data, such as the Confidence Profile

Method (14), use Bayesian methods to calculate posterior probability distributions for effects of interest. Bayesian statistics are based on the principle that each observation or set of observations should be viewed in conjunction with a prior probability describing the prior knowledge of the phenomenon of interest (15). The new observations alter this prior probability to generate a posterior probability. Traditional meta-analysis assumes that nothing is known about the magnitude of the treatment effect before randomized trials are performed. In Bayesian terms, the prior probability distribution is noninformative. Bayesian approaches may also allow the incorporation of indirect evidence in generating prior distributions (14) and may be particularly helpful in situations in which few data from randomized studies exist (16). Bayesian analyses may also be used to account for the uncertainty introduced by estimating the between-study variance in the random-effects model, leading to more appropriate estimates and predictions of treatment efficacy (17).

Exploring and Explaining Heterogeneity

The next important issue is whether the common estimate obtained in the previous step is robust. Sensitivity analyses determine whether the common estimate is influenced by changes in the assumptions and in the protocol for combining the data.

A comparison of the results of fixed- and random-effects models is one such sensitivity analysis (18). Generally, the random-effects model produces wider CIs than does the fixed-effects model, and the level of statistical significance may therefore be different depending on the model used. The pooled point estimate per se is less likely to be affected, although exceptions are possible (19).

Other sensitivity analyses may include the examination of the residuals and the chi-square components (13) and assessment of the effect of deleting each study in turn. Statistically significant results that depend on a single study may require further exploration.

Cumulative Meta-Analysis

Cumulative meta-analysis is another approach for assessing the impact of each study (20); it is the opposite of the stepwise deletion. In cumulative meta-analysis, studies are sequentially pooled by adding one study at a time in a prespecified order (21). One possible order is according to the dates these studies were conducted or published. Cumulative meta-analysis can help determine whether the pooled estimate has been robust over time and can also determine the point in time when statistical significance was reached for a pooled result. When the order is the year of publication, cumulative meta-analysis can be seen as a form of Bayesian inference. The prior probability (the prior belief) is generated by the pooled results of all prior studies, and the posterior probability is derived by adding the results of the new study to the results of the others (21).

Meta-Regression

Further sensitivity analyses are generally dictated by the nature and the specifics of the question that the meta-analysis tries to answer and by the possible reasons that can be identified to explain heterogeneity. One such computational procedure, commonly referred to as meta-regression, involves the statistical assessment of whether specific factors (covariates) influence the magnitude of the point estimate of the treatment effect across studies (22). Meta-regression results are generally reported as slope coefficients with CIs. The covariates of interest may describe study or patient characteristics. These characteristics may be common for all patients in each study (for example, the specific route of administration of the experimental drug used in each study) or they may be average values representative of the studied cohort (such as the mean age of the patients). Averages of covariates measured at the patient level require cautious interpretation because the aggregate values may not adequately represent important minorities of patients (23-25).

Some covariates are ubiquitous, such as study sample size, study result variance, and control rate of events (the percentage of patients with an event of interest in the control group). Other covariates may be problem-specific. Often, information on covariates may not be uniformly collected or reported across all studies, and analyses involving these covariates may therefore not be useful. A variety of statistical methods, including weighted least-squares, logistic regression, and hierarchical models, can be used for meta-regression analyses (22, 26-28).

Figure 9.1 summarizes the three previous steps, which define the core of a meta-analysis. It shows that estimating, deciding whether to ignore, incorporating, exploring, and explaining heterogeneity are the key aims of the quantitative methods for synthesizing data from different studies.

Subgroup Analysis

Subgroup analyses may be useful for addressing particular questions when data for different subgroups of patients are available from each study (29). Combining specific subgroup data across studies follows the principles described above and may provide further insight into heterogeneity. Subgroup analyses in the retrospective setting of most meta-analyses are post hoc exercises and should be interpreted with caution, lest they turn into "fishing expeditions." An especially pernicious approach occurs when the data are divided into multiple subgroups on the basis of combinations of characteristics (such as age and dose) and differential treatment effects are claimed within very small subdivisions. Such interactions among subgroups are

unlikely to describe the truth when derived from aggregated data.

Lack of uniform reporting of the data necessary for subgroup analyses across trials poses an additional problem. Thus, subgroup analyses should best be used as hypothesis-generating tools (22), although important observations may sometimes be made (30).

Assessing the Potential for Bias

The assessment of potential bias should always be part of a meta-analysis. Some issues relevant to this were discussed in Chapters 7 and 8 (1, 2). Two major sources of bias for meta-analysis are the failure to find all of the studies performed in the clinical domain and the uncertain reliability of poor-quality studies.

Publication Bias

Studies with negative results are more likely to remain unpublished because investigators or the peer reviewers and editors are not enthusiastic about publishing "negative" information (31-33). The chances of not being published are probably greater if the negative study is small and nonrandomized (34). Some studies may be impossible to retrieve and include in a meta-analysis despite a thorough search of potential databases. Publication bias is difficult to eliminate, but some statistical procedures may be helpful in detecting its presence. An inverted funnel plot (35) is sometimes used to visually explore the possibility that publication bias is present (Figure 9.2). This method uses a scatterplot of studies that relates the magnitude of the treatment effect to the weight of the study. An inverted, funnel-shaped, symmetrical appearance of dots suggests that no study has been left out, whereas an asymmetrical appearance suggests the presence of publication bias. Formal computational approaches to test for, assess the extent of, and correct publication bias have also been described (36-39).

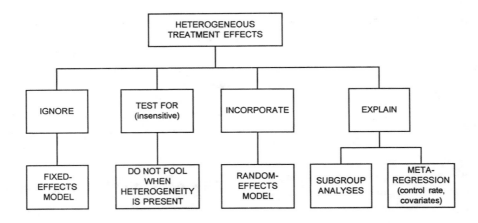

Figure 9.1 Methodologic choices and their implications in dealing with heterogeneous data in a meta-analysis.

Quality

Study quality was discussed in detail in Chapter 8. Investigators have proposed incorporating quality scores into meta-analyses on the basis of checklists of study design components (40-43). To date, no scale has been proven to correlate consistently with treatment efficacy (44). Beyond the generic features of study design and conduct, general quality-scoring systems may have to be supplemented or replaced with more problem-specific quality items for each particular meta-analysis (45). Empirical investigations have shown that studies of worse quality may overestimate treatment effects because they inadequately conceal treatment allocation and use inadequate blinding (46).

Presenting the Results

The results of meta-analyses are typically presented in a graphic form (Figure 9.3) that shows the point estimates and their CIs. This presentation aims to convey an impression of the results of the individual studies, to convey the extent of heterogeneity, and to report the pooled estimate. Meta-regression analyses may be depicted by plots in which the value of the covariate of interest is shown on the horizontal axis

and the magnitude of the treatment effect is shown on the vertical axis (48). It is also important to report results from sensitivity analyses on key issues and comparison between fixed-effects and random-effects methods of pooling data when their results are different. When appropriate, reporting the NNT helps translate the results into a more clinically meaningful metric (3).

Other Types of Data and Methods

Meta-Analysis of Diagnostic Tests

An important application of meta-analysis is the combination of sensitivity and specificity data of diagnostic tests across different studies (49). Using weighted linear regression to generate a summary receiver-operating characteristics (ROC) curve has been proposed as a way to avoid the underestimation of test performance that results when the correlation between sensitivity and specificity is ignored (50). An ROC curve is a plot of the percentage of true-positive results (the sensitivity of the test) against the percentage of false-positive results (1—specificity) and thus represents the tradeoff between these two test characteristics.

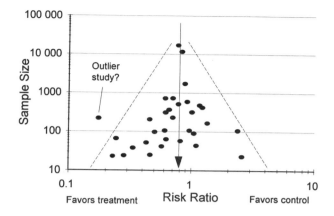

Figure 9.2 An inverted funnel plot to detect publication bias. This example used data from a meta-analysis of intravenous streptokinase for acute myocardial infarction (20). The risk ratio for the mortality reduction in each study is plotted against the weight of the study, represented by the sample size. A symmetric triangle is fitted around the pooled estimate (*arrow*) so that it encompasses most of the studies. If small "negative" trials with large variance have been left unpublished, the plot will be asymmetrical: Small studies will show very large estimates of the treatment effect compared with larger studies that have more conservative results. A symmetrical plot provides reassuring evidence that the treatment effect is similar in studies of small and large variance, whereas an asymmetrical plot suggests possible publication bias. This plot reveals that there are fewer small studies (involving 10 to 100 participants) with risk ratios greater than 0.8 than there are small studies with risk ratios less than 0.8, whereas the numbers of medium and large studies are fairly symmetric. These results suggest that some small studies with negative findings were not published. Outlier studies may also be readily identified by using this plot.

Meta-Analysis of Other Nonrandomized, Uncontrolled Data

Uncontrolled cohort data can also be combined by using meta-analytic techniques. The principles are the same as those described for randomized data. However, greater care is needed in the conduct of the analysis and interpretation of the results when nonrandomized and uncontrolled data are used because these data are more likely to be biased. Of particular interest is the synthesis of dose-response data across different studies that investigate the effect of increasing values of a potential etiologic factor on an outcome of interest (for example, exposure to environmental tobacco smoke and the occurrence of lung cancer) (17, 51-53).

Meta-Analysis of Individual Patient Data

Most meta-analyses are based on group data as reported in the literature, but researchers occasionally make the effort to collect the detailed outcomes and risk factor data for the individual patients involved in each of several studies. These data can be used in survival analyses and multivariate regression analyses. Meta-analysis of individual patient data is more expensive and time-consuming than meta-analysis of grouped data, and it requires the coordination of large teams of investigators and a robust protocol (54). Nevertheless, if possible, meta-analysis of individual patient data may represent the highest step in the hierarchy of evidence (55).

Conclusions

By quantitatively summarizing a collection of data from clinical studies, meta-analysis provides collective results of a kind that no individual study can offer. Meta-analysis is a relatively new discipline in clinical medicine. As might be expected, discrepancies between the results of large trials and meta-analyses of smaller trials (19), as well as differences in the results of meta-analyses addressing the same topic, do occur (56, 57). New quantitative methods are being devel-

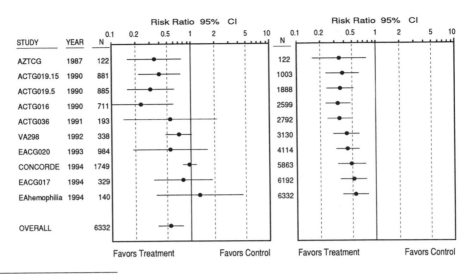

Figure 9.3 Standard meta-analysis and cumulative meta-analysis. *Left,* A standard meta-analysis plot of the risk ratios for progression to AIDS or death in a comparison of early therapy with zidovudine (treatment group) or deferred therapy with zidovudine (control group) (47). The point estimates for the risk ratio of each study and the pooled point estimate are shown by the points, and the horizontal lines show the CIs, typically 95% CIs. *N* is the number of patients in the study. The studies are ordered according to year of publication. As a standard convention, a risk ratio of less than 1 denotes a reduction in the number of events in the treated compared with the control group. *Right,* The results of a cumulative meta-analysis of the same data. *N* is the number of patients in the clinical trials. The points and lines represent the point estimates and the 95% CIs of the pooled results after the inclusion of each additional study in the calculations. The CIs typically narrow with the addition of more studies unless substantial heterogeneity exists.

oped, and investigators have addressed these important issues (58-60). Synthesis of the data from many individual studies requires sound, rigorous, quantitative methods, and the results of such syntheses should be interpreted with appropriate caution; meta-analysis is not a "magic" solution to the problem of scientific evidence and cannot replace clinical reasoning (61). In addition, reliable meta-analysis requires consistent, high-quality reporting of the primary data from individual studies; the need for such reporting cannot be overstated (62, 63).

Key Points To Remember

• Systematic reviews often use complex statistical methods to synthesize and interpret data, and an understanding of their basic principles is important in interpreting their results.

• Quantitative synthesis cannot replace sound clinical reasoning; combining poor-quality or overly biased data or data that do not make sense is likely to produce unreliable results.

• When appropriate, combining studies to obtain a common estimate can increase the statistical power for discovering treatment efficacy and can increase the precision of the estimate.

• Sensitivity analyses should be performed to determine the robustness of conclusions.

• Patients, clinical settings, and treatment responses are expected to vary across trials that have studied the same problem. Insight into reasons for the heterogeneity of trial results may often be as important as or even more important than obtaining aggregate results.

Glossary

Bayesian inference: A statistical discipline that addresses how a prior estimate should be modified in the light of knowledge gained from new studies.

Cumulative meta-analysis: A method whereby the combined point estimate of an effect is sequentially computed by adding one study at a time in a prespecified order.

Fixed-effects model: A model that assumes that all studies are studying the same true effect and that variability is due to random error only.

Heterogeneity: The diversity that exists between studies. It may be due to identifiable factors or statistical factors, or both, especially the component that cannot be explained by random error.

Meta-regression: A regression analysis in which individual sets of data (studies) are used as the unit of observation.

Random-effects model: A model that assumes that the true effect differs among studies and therefore must be represented by a distribution of values instead of a single value.

Receiver-operating characteristic curve: A plot of the characteristics of a diagnostic test. It depicts the tradeoff between the sensitivity and the specificity of the test.

Acknowledgments: The authors thank Drs. Andrew Oxman and Larry V. Hedges for their reviews of and valuable comments on the manuscript and thank the clinical reviewer, Norman J. Wilder.

Grant Support: In part by grants R01 HS07782 and R01 HS 08532 from the Agency for Health Care Policy and Research (Drs. Lau and Schmid) and grant T32 AI07389 from the National Institutes of Health (Dr. Ioannidis).

References

1. **Counsell C.** Formulating questions and locating primary studies for inclusion in systematic reviews. Ann Intern Med. 1997;127:380-7.
2. **Meade MO, Richardson WS.** Selecting and appraising studies for a systematic review. Ann Intern Med. 1997;127:531-7.
3. **McQuay HJ, Moore RA.** Using numerical results from systematic reviews in clinical practice. Ann Intern Med. 1997;126:712-20.
4. **Sinclair JC, Bracken MB.** Clinically useful measures of effect in binary analyses of randomized trials. J Clin Epidemiol. 1994;47:881-90.
5. **Cooper H, Hedges LV.** The Handbook of Research Synthesis. New York: Russell Sage Foundation; 1994.
6. **Fleiss JL.** Statistical Methods for Rates and Proportions. 2d ed. New York: J Wiley; 1981:161-5.
7. **Mantel N, Haenszel W.** Statistical aspects of the analysis of data from retrospective studies of disease. J Natl Cancer Inst. 1959;22:719-48.
8. **Laird NM, Mosteller F.** Some statistical methods for combining experimental results. Int J Technol Assess Health Care. 1990;6:5-30.
9. **Yusuf S, Peto R, Lewis J, Collins R, Sleight P.** Beta blockade during and after myocardial infarction: an overview of the randomized trials. Prog Cardiovasc Dis. 1985;27:335-71.
10. **Greenland S, Salvan A.** Bias in the one-step method for pooling study results. Stat Med. 1990;9:247-52.
11. **Fleiss JL.** The statistical basis of meta-analysis. Stat Methods Med Res. 1993;2:121-45.
12. **DerSimonian R, Laird N.** Meta-analysis in clinical trials. Control Clin Trials. 1986;7:177-88.
13. **Hedges LV, Olkin I.** Statistical Methods for Meta-Analysis. Orlando: Academic Pr; 1985.
14. **Eddy DM, Hasselblad V, Schacter RD.** Meta-Analysis by the Confidence Profile Method: The Statistical Synthesis of Evidence. New York: Academic Pr; 1991.
15. **Gelman A, Carlin JB, Stern HS, Rubin DB.** Bayesian Data Analysis. London: Chapman & Hall; 1995:148-54.
16. **Lilford RJ, Thornton JG, Braunholtz D.** Clinical trials and rare diseases: a way out of a conundrum. BMJ. 1995;311:1621-5.
17. **Dumouchel W.** Meta-analysis for dose-response models. Stat Med. 1995;14:679-85.
18. **Berlin JA, Laird NM, Sacks HS, Chalmers TC.** A comparison of statistical methods for combining event rates from clinical trials. Stat Med. 1989;8:141-51.
19. **Borzak S, Ridker PM.** Discordance between meta-analyses and large-scale randomized, controlled trials. Examples from the management of acute myocardial infarction. Ann Intern Med. 1995;123:873-7.
20. **Lau J, Antman EM, Jimenez-Silva J, Kupelnick B, Mosteller F, Chalmers TC.** Cumulative meta-analysis of therapeutic trials for myocardial infarction. N Engl J Med. 1992;327:248-54.
21. **Lau J, Schmid CH, Chalmers TC.** Cumulative meta-analysis of clinical trials builds evidence for exemplary medical care. J Clin Epidemiol. 1995;48:45-57.
22. **Berlin JA, Antman EM.** Advantages and limitations of metaanalytic regressions of clinical trials data. Online J Curr Clin Trials. 4 June 1994: Doc. No. 134.
23. **Morgenstern H.** Uses of ecologic analysis in epidemiologic research. Am J Public Health. 1982;72:1336-44.
24. **Langbein LI, Lichtman AJ.** Ecological Inference. Beverly Hills, CA: Sage; 1978. (Sage University Paper Series on Quantitative Applications in the Social Sciences. Series no. 07-010.)

25. **Greenland S, Robins J.** Invited commentary: ecologic studies-biases, misconceptions, and counterexamples. Am J Epidemiol. 1994;139:747-60.

26. **McIntosh M.** The population risk as an explanatory variable in research synthesis of clinical trials. Stat Med. 1996;15:1713-28.

27. **Morris CN, Normand SL.** Hierarchical models for combining information and for meta-analyses. In: Bernardo JM, Berger JO, Dawid AP, Smith AF. Bayesian Statistics 4. New York: Oxford Univ Pr; 1992.

28. **Smith TC, Spiegelhalter DJ, Thomas A.** Bayesian approaches to random-effects meta-analysis: a comparative study. Stat Med. 1995;14:2685-99.

29. **Oxman AD, Guyatt GH.** A consumer's guide to subgroup analyses. Ann Intern Med. 1992;116:78-84.

30. **Michels KB, Rosner BA.** Data trawling: to fish or not to fish. Lancet. 1996;348:1152-3.

31. **Dickersin K, Chan S, Chalmers TC, Sacks HS, Smith H Jr.** Publication bias and clinical trials. Control Clin Trials. 1987;8:343-53.

32. **Dickersin K.** The existence of publication bias and risk factors for its occurrence. JAMA. 1990;263:1385-9.

33. **Begg CB.** Publication bias. In: Cooper H, Hedges L, eds. The Handbook of Research Synthesis. New York: Russell Sage Foundation; 1994.

34. **Easterbrook PJ, Berlin JA, Gopalan R, Matthews DR.** Publication bias in clinical research. Lancet. 1991;337:867-72.

35. **Light RJ, Pillemer DB.** Summing up: the science of reviewing research. Cambridge, MA: Harvard Univ Pr; 1984.

36. **Begg CB, Mazumdar M.** Operating characteristics of a rank correlation test for publication bias. Biometrics. 1994;50:1088-101.

37. **Dear KB, Begg CB.** An approach for assessing publication bias prior to performing a meta-analysis. Statistical Science. 1992;7:237-45.

38. **Hedges LV.** Modeling publication selection effects in random effects models in meta-analysis. Statistical Science. 1992;7:246-55.

39. **Vevea JL, Hedges LV.** A general linear model for estimating effect size in the presence of publication bias. Psychometrika. 1995;60:419-35.

40. **Chalmers TC, Smith H Jr, Blackburn B, Silverman B, Schroeder B, Reitman D, et al.** A method for assessing the quality of a randomized control trial. Control Clin Trials. 1981;2:31-49.

41. **Mulrow CD, Linn WD, Gaul MK, Pugh JA.** Assessing quality of a diagnostic test evaluation. J Gen Intern Med. 1989;4:288-95.

42. **Detsky AS, Naylor CD, O'Rourke K, McGeer AJ, L'Abbe KA.** Incorporating variations in the quality of individual randomized trials into meta-analysis. J Clin Epidemiol. 1992;45:255-65.

43. **Moher D, Jadad AR, Nichol G, Penman M, Tugwell P, Walsh S.** Assessing the quality of randomized controlled trials: an annotated bibliography of scales and checklists. Control Clin Trials. 1995;16:62-73.

44. **Emerson JD, Burdick E, Hoaglin DC, Mosteller F, Chalmers TC.** An empirical study of the possible relation of treatment differences to quality scores in controlled randomized clinical trials. Control Clin Trials. 1990;11:339-52.

45. **Greenland S.** Invited commentary: a critical look at some popular meta-analytic methods. Am J Epidemiol. 1994;140:290-6.

46. **Schultz KF, Chalmers I, Hayes RJ, Altman DG.** Empirical evidence of bias. Dimension of methodological quality associated with estimates of treatment effects in controlled trials. JAMA. 1995;273:408-12.

47. **Ioannidis JP, Cappelleri JC, Lau J, Skolnik PR, Melville B, Chalmers TC, et al.** Early or deferred zidovudine therapy in HIV-infected patients without an AIDS-defining illness. Ann Intern Med. 1995;122:856-66.

48. **Holme I.** Relation of coronary heart disease incidence and total mortality to plasma cholesterol reduction in randomised trials: use of meta-analysis. Br Heart J. 1993;69(1 Suppl):S42-7.

49. **Irwig L, Tosteson AN, Gatsonis C, Lau J, Colditz G, Chalmers TC, et al.** Guidelines for meta-analyses evaluating diagnostic tests. Ann Intern Med. 1994;120:667-76.

50. **Moses LE, Shapiro D, Littenberg B.** Combining independent studies of a diagnostic test into a summary ROC curve: data-analytic approaches and some additional considerations. Stat Med. 1993;12:1293-316.

51. **Tweedie RL, Mengersen KL.** Meta-analytic approaches to dose-response relationships, with application in studies of lung cancer and exposure to environmental tobacco smoke. Stat Med. 1995;14:545-69.

52. **Greenland S, Longnecker MP.** Methods for trend estimation from summarized dose-response data, with applications to meta-analysis. Am J Epidemiol. 1992;135:1301-9.

53. **Smith SJ, Caudill SP, Steinberg KK, Thacker SB.** On combining dose-response data from epidemiological studies by meta-analysis. Stat Med. 1995;14:531-44.

54. **Stewart LA, Clarke MJ.** Practical methodology of meta-analyses (overviews) using updated individual patient data. Cochrane Working Group. Stat Med. 1995;14:2057-79.

55. **Olkin I.** Statistical and theoretical considerations in meta-analysis. J Clin Epidemiol. 1995;48:133-46.

56. **Cook DJ, Witt LG, Cook RJ, Guyatt GH.** Stress ulcer prophylaxis in the critically ill: a meta-analysis. Am J Med. 1991;91:519-27.

57. **Tryba M.** Prophylaxis of stress ulcer bleeding. A meta-analysis. J Clin Gastroenterol. 1991:13(Suppl 2):S44-55.

58. **Villar J, Carroli G, Belizan JM.** Predictive ability of meta-analyses of randomised controlled trials. Lancet. 1995;345:772-6.

59. **Cappelleri JC, Ioannidis JP, Schmid CH, de Ferranti SD, Aubert M, Chalmers TC, et al.** Large trials vs meta-analysis of smaller trials: how do their results compare? JAMA. 1996;276:1332-8.

60. **Cook DJ, Reeve BK, Guyatt GH, Heyland DK, Griffith LE, Buckingham L, et al.** Stress ulcer prophylaxis in critically ill patients. Resolving discordant meta-analyses. JAMA. 1996;275:308-14.

61. **Ioannidis JP, Lau J.** On meta-analyses of meta-analyses [Letter]. Lancet. 1996;348:756.

62. **Altman DG.** Better reporting of randomised controlled trials: the CONSORT statement. BMJ. 1996;313:570-1.

63. **Begg C, Cho M, Eastwood S, Horton R, Moher D, Olkin I, et al.** Improving the quality of reporting of randomized controlled trials. The CONSORT statement. JAMA. 1996;276:637-9.

Chapter 10

Integrating Heterogeneous Pieces of Evidence in Systematic Reviews

Cynthia Mulrow, MD, MSc; Peter Langhorne, PhD, MRCP; and Jeremy Grimshaw, MBChB, MRCGP

Researchers preparing systematic reviews often encounter various types of evidence that can generally be categorized as direct or indirect. The former directly relates an exposure, diagnostic strategy, or therapeutic intervention to the occurrence of a principal health outcome. Evidence is indirect if two or more bodies of evidence are required to relate the exposure, diagnostic strategy, or intervention to the principal health outcome.

Heterogeneity of data sources complicates integration of both direct and indirect evidence. Participants in different studies may have a wide spectrum of baseline risk and sociodemographic and cultural characteristics. A variety of formulations and intensities of exposures, diagnostic strategies, and interventions, as well as diversity in the selection and definition of control groups, may be encountered. Outcome measures may be different, and similar outcomes may be measured or reported differently. Heterogeneity of study designs and of methodologic features and quality within a given design may be found. The effective integration of direct and indirect evidence requires development of explicit models that serve as analytic frameworks for linking the important pieces of evidence. A model can be viewed as a series of "subquestions," with each important subquestion warranting a systematic review. Several subjective and quantitative methods can then be used to integrate the evidence. Tabular displays of major findings and strength of evidence for each subquestion can help reviewers, patients, and providers to integrate the differing research findings and draw reasonable conclusions. Various quantitative techniques, such as decision analysis and the confidence profile method, are also available. No single integration approach is clearly superior, none obviates uncertainty, and all underscore the role of careful judgment in integrating evidence.

Previous chapters have described systematic reviews and how to find them (1, 2), discussed their role in practice and educational settings (3-6), and outlined important aspects of their conduct (7-9). This chapter addresses a particularly challenging problem in conducting systematic reviews: integration of different types of evidence within a single review. We present strategies for integrating evidence from various primary studies that were conducted with different objectives, protocols, and designs. These strategies may be useful in a variety of situations in which heterogeneous evidence is used (for example, clinical decisions, decision analysis, economic analysis, practice guidelines, and health policy formulations). The strategies are intended primarily for reviewers who address broad questions (for example, reviewers interested in producing evidence-based guidelines). The strategies may also help reviewers with focused questions when the data available on a topic are particularly heterogeneous.

We consider the following specific questions: 1) How can reviewers classify and structure heterogeneous research evidence? 2) What factors complicate integration of heterogeneous research evidence? 3) What strategies help integrate heterogeneous research evidence?

Classifying and Structuring Research Evidence

Just as any scientific inquiry moves from concrete observations to abstract concepts, reviewers must move from samples of data (individual pieces of evidence) to more general conclusions (10). This process involves drawing together multiple pieces of evidence into a unified whole by categorizing and ordering data (11). An important first step is to classify evidence as direct or indirect.

Direct evidence directly relates an exposure, diagnostic strategy, or therapeutic intervention to the occurrence of a principal health outcome (12). Principal health outcomes are those relevant to the patient, such as symptoms, loss of function, and death (13). Whether or not a study provides direct evidence depends on methodologic design and the outcomes studied. For example, some randomized, controlled trials that compared diuretic and β-blocker regimens with no therapy or placebo in hypertensive adults have directly shown that these therapies decrease cardiovascular morbidity and mortality (14). Other trials comparing antihypertensive agents have shown decreases in blood pressure (a surrogate outcome) but have not directly demonstrated effects on cardiovascular morbidity and mortality (the principal outcomes).

Evidence is indirect if two or more bodies of evidence are required to relate the exposure or intervention of interest to the principal health outcome (12). Thus, one body of evidence may relate exercise (the intervention) to lower-extremity strength (an intermediate outcome), and another may relate lower-extremity strength to the probability of falls (the health outcome of principal interest); neither one alone directly relates exercise to falls. Other examples are intervention strategies with several substitutes, particularly when the various substitutes have been evaluated in different types of studies. For example, pravastatin, a 3-hydroxy-3-methylglutaryl-coenzyme A reductase inhibitor, has been shown to decrease low-density lipoprotein cholesterol levels and cardiovascular morbidity and mortality in men with moderate hypercholesterolemia and no history of myocardial infarction (primary prevention) (15). Several of these inhibitors, including pravastatin, simvastatin, and fluvastatin, have been shown to decrease cardiovascular morbidity or mortality in persons with hypercholesterolemia and history of myocardial infarction (secondary prevention) (16, 17, Oral presentation of the

Lipoprotein and Coronary Atherosclerosis Study at American Heart Association Meeting, Anaheim, California, November 1996). Taken together, these data provide indirect rather than direct evidence that all 3-hydroxy-3-methylglutaryl-coenzyme A reductase inhibitors are effective in the primary prevention of cardiovascular disease.

Much evidence about health care is indirect. The synthesis of indirect evidence or of pieces of direct evidence requires the creation of models that relate exposures or diagnostic or intervention strategies to principal health outcomes. Conceptually, this involves 1) identifying links that connect the exposures, diagnostic strategies, or interventions to principal health outcomes; 2) analyzing the evidence that pertains to each link; and 3) combining the links (12). In essence, this approach breaks a complex problem into a series of smaller problems and formally theorizes the relations among those problems. Such models are often called evidence models. They provide reviewers with an analytic framework that clarifies the cause or natural history of a health problem, the sequence of intermediate effects that an exposure or diagnostic or intervention strategy must pass through to reach certain primary outcomes, and the range of potential adverse effects that need consideration (18, 19).

Factors Complicating Integration of Evidence

Regardless of whether reviewers are synthesizing direct or indirect evidence, many factors can modify etiologic and prognostic associations, diagnostic accuracy, and therapeutic effectiveness. Study participants are often drawn from various settings and have a wide spectrum of baseline risk, disease severity, and sociodemographic and cultural characteristics. Exposures, diagnostic strategies, interventions, and comparison groups have varying formulations and intensities. Different outcome measures are used in different studies, and similar outcomes are measured or reported differently. Various study designs are used (Table 10.1), and heterogeneity of methodologic features occurs within a given design (Table 10.2).

Heterogeneity of research evidence may concurrently exist at one or more levels. A review of several randomized, controlled trials that tested whether a particular drug class resulted in improved survival in similar groups of patients may be complicated only by judgments on the degree of homogeneity of the different drugs within the class. In practice, heterogeneity of only one factor in a given study or group of studies (for example, different drugs within a class) is relatively rare; several sources of complexity are usually present. For example, a recent systematic review of the effectiveness of stroke units included evidence from both randomized and nonrandomized controlled clinical trials; these trials evaluated different models of stroke units, used different patient inclusion criteria, and had various outcome measures (20). Systematic reviews that examined studies of methods for implementing clinical guidelines have included multifaceted management interventions directed toward different clinical conditions; systematic reviews of the effica-

Table 10.1   Potential Sources of Research Evidence

Primary studies in humans
  Randomized, controlled trials
  Nonrandomized, controlled trials
  Cohort or longitudinal studies
  Case–control studies
  Cross-sectional descriptions and surveys
  Case series and reports
Nonhuman studies
  In vitro (laboratory) studies
  Animal studies
Syntheses
  Systematic reviews, including meta-analyses
  Decision and economic analyses

Table 10.2 Examples of Important Methodologic Features Associated with Different Types of Studies

Type of Study	Methodologic Characteristics That Reduce Bias
Intervention	Randomized trial
	Controlled trial
	Blinding of outcome assessment
	Blinding of intervention assignment
	Complete follow-up of randomly assigned participants
Disease association	
Cohort study	Defined (inception) cohort
	Objective outcome criteria used
	Blinding of outcome assessment
	Complete follow-up of recruited participants
	Adjustment for confounding factors
Case–control study	Random sampling procedure to recruit participants
	Appropriate source of controls
	Small number of nonrespondents
	Close matching of control group
	Reliability and blinding of assessments
	Adjustment for confounding factors
Prognosis	
Cohort study	See under "disease association"
Diagnosis	
Comparative study	Acceptable reference (gold) standard
	Independent reading of results of test and reference standard
	Verification with reference standard in all patients
	Random allocation (or complete allocation) of patients to tests

cy of continuing medical education examined studies of a variety of educational activities among different groups of health care professionals working in different health care settings (21, 22). A comprehensive review evaluating the association between cigarette smoking and lung cancer might integrate evidence from laboratory studies of genetic mutations with evidence from case-control and prospective studies of cancer in animals and humans.

Heterogeneity is a double-edged sword. On the positive side, it may allow reviewers to examine consistency of findings across studies of various types and their applicability in a variety of patients and settings (that is, it may increase generalizability). It may also allow a more comprehensive picture of feasibility, acceptability, benefits, and harms associated with particular formulations of a diagnostic or therapeutic strategy. On the negative side, it may introduce ambiguity into the synthesis of evidence. Researchers conducting systematic reviews may be required to make judgments about the relevance of the heterogeneity, the legitimacy and relative uncertainty of particular pieces of evidence, the importance of missing evidence, the soundness of the model for linking the evidence, and the appropriateness of conducting a quantitative summary.

Strategies for Integrating Heterogeneous Evidence

Linking Multiple Pieces of Evidence

Reviewers addressing broad questions that involve linkages among multiple bodies of both indirect and direct evidence need to use explicitly defined models. An example of a model that was used to guide a systematic review of screening for hearing impairment in elderly persons is given in Figure 10.1 (23). The model was based on preset criteria for evaluating screening programs (24). Frameworks for constructing models of causality, prognosis, effectiveness of diagnostic and intervention strategies, and specific relationships between surrogate and clinically meaningful outcomes are also available (12, 13, 18, 25, 26). An example of a complex framework for assessing benefits and harms of a particular therapy is given in Figure 10.2. Each link in

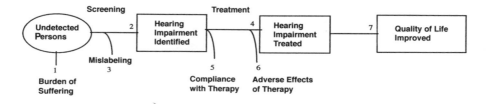

Figure 10.1 Model examining rationale for screening for hearing impairment. The following are focused questions associated with some of the linkages shown. *Linkage 2:* What is the accuracy of screening tests (whispered voice, tuning fork, finger rub, questionnaires, audioscope) for identifying elderly patients with hearing impairments? *Linkage 3:* What adverse effects from mislabeling result from measuring hearing impairment in elderly patients with previously undetected hearing impairment? *Linkage 4:* Does treating hearing-impaired elderly patients by using hearing aids improve the acuity of hearing?

a model represents a subquestion for which a systematic review could be conducted. In some instances, direct evidence that obviates the need to address certain intermediate linkages may be available. Reviewers select important linkages and perform a series of pertinent systematic reviews, each with a well-formulated question, specified inclusion criteria, explicit searching and selection techniques, and method of critical appraisal. Evidence tables for each subquestion can be developed (Table 10.3). These can be accompanied by narrative summaries that identify the direction, magnitude, significance, and uncertainty of effects and highlight major issues affecting the applicability and validity of data. For some subquestions, meta-analyses may be possible. Likewise, for some subquestions on prognosis, diagnosis, or therapy, the strength or level of available evidence may be ranked by using criteria that emphasize methodologic rigor and avoidance of bias (27-32).

The techniques for integrating and interpreting multiple types and units of evidence are evolving. Current methods include subjective as well as quantitative approaches (33). One subjective approach is to create a tabular display or balance sheet that lists the major findings (such as the direction, magnitude, and uncertainty of effects) and strength of evidence for each subquestion. The goal is to condense important information into a display that

can be grasped both visually and mentally (34). Reviewers then use the tabular displays as structures for integrating a mixture of research findings and for drawing conclusions. Patients and their providers can also use the displays to integrate evidence and make their own personalized decisions. Several potential pitfalls need to be considered, however, when global interpretations and judgments are made on the basis of balance sheets. These pitfalls include overrelying on single outcomes; using statistical significance as a proxy for the clinical impact (effect size) of an outcome, ignoring the actual magnitude of effects and the degree of uncertainty associated with those effects, failure to differentiate surrogate from clinically meaningful outcomes, and retreating to such generalities as "cancer is bad, so any intervention that combats it is worthwhile" (18).

Another subjective yet explicit approach is to base integration and conclusions on a limited number of important variables. The U.S. Preventive Services Task Force, for example, subjectively integrated research on preventive care strategies on the basis of three criteria: burden of suffering from the target condition; characteristics of the prevention strategy, such as feasibility; and demonstrated effectiveness of the strategy determined by considering the rigor of available evidence. By using this three-pronged approach, the Task Force concluded that there was good evidence (grade A) to recommend screening for cervical cancer with Papanicolaou testing even though no data from randomized, controlled trials directly show the clinical benefits of screening with this technique (35).

More singular emphasis on the methodologic strength or level of evidence can be used to draw conclusions (29). An important pitfall to avoid in this approach is confusing lack of high-level evidence with evidence against a particular strategy. Absence of proof is not proof of absence. Moreover, a single item of high-level evidence may be available for a particular diagnostic strategy

or therapeutic intervention; although no high-level evidence exists for alternative strategies, many pieces of indirect evidence may at the same time suggest the superiority of the alternative strategies.

A variety of quantitative models is available for linking intermediate events and several pieces of evidence together in sequence. Formal decision analyses are quantitative models that use explicit paths to connect decisions to intermediate and final outcomes. The paths represent a series of actions and events, beginning with an initial choice node and ending in outcomes

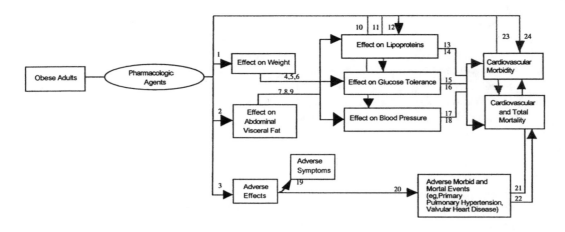

Figure 10.2 An evidence model for the pharmacologic treatment of obesity. The following are focused questions associated with some of the linkages shown. *Linkage 7:* Does the effect of pharmacologic agents on abdominal or visceral fat lead to improved lipoprotein levels? *Linkage 8:* Does the effect of pharmacologic agents on abdominal or visceral fat affect control of blood sugar? *Linkage 9:* Does the effect of pharmacologic agents on abdominal or visceral fat affect control of blood pressure? *Linkage 10:* Does pharmacologic treatment of obesity affect control of blood pressure independently of its effect on weight or abdominal or visceral fat?

Table 10.3   Example of Items To Include in Evidence Table*

Study, Year	Condition of Interest	Sample Size	Participant Characteristics			Setting	Basic Design	Patients Blinded?	Outcome Assessment Blinded?
			Mean Age	Men					
		n	*y*	*%*					
Smith, 2000	Better ear threshold threshold ≥40 dB at 2000 Hz	1340	79	40	Primary care clinic	Randomized, controlled trial	No	No

*Hypothetical example of trial addressing efficacy of hearing aids for hearing-impaired elderly persons.
†HHIE = Hearing Handicap Inventory in the Elderly Questionnaire, which measures emotional and social effects of hearing loss (score range, 0–100).

that can be weighted to reflect patient preferences or utilities (36-38). Probabilities of all possible outcomes, which are ideally estimated by using individual systematic reviews, are combined to determine the optimal course of action. Advanced stochastic modeling techniques, such as Markov chains, state-transition models, and difference equations, can be used to analyze particularly complex multidirectional relations (39). A relatively new technique, the confidence profile method, allows analysis of evidence involving mixed comparisons (for example, drawing conclusions about A compared with B on the basis of evidence about A compared with C and C compared with B) (40). Adjustments for prior probabilities, biases, and relative uncertainties that are pertinent to particular pieces of evidence can be incorporated into these models. All of these quantitative techniques have limitations because they rely on many assumptions; require special computational tools, software, and statistical expertise; and usually are not transparent to users of evidence.

Addressing Heterogeneity in Single Bodies of Evidence

Even reviewers who address focused questions are challenged by heterogeneity. One way of dealing with this problem is to use narrow inclusion criteria. For example, reviewers may review only studies that report a particular outcome. This approach ensures a more uniform data set that may limit ambiguity. The drawbacks of such narrow focus include the risk for losing valuable information and the possibility of introducing bias in favor of studies that report outcomes in a particular way (41). Some reviewers restrict reviews to particular study designs or, even more severely, to particular study designs with certain methodologic characteristics (for example, double-blind, randomized, controlled trials rather than randomized, controlled trials). Although these approaches may limit bias, we still do not fully understand all of the factors that influence the validity of most study designs; thus, we may receive a false sense of assurance from the use of such restrictive techniques. Furthermore, the quality of studies is a continuum, and evidence from well-conducted studies with "weaker" designs may be more robust than evidence from poorly conducted studies with more "rigorous" designs.

Quantitative methods for coping with heterogeneity include sensitivity analyses that explore the effect of grouping data in a variety of ways (9). A good example is a recent meta-analysis of oral contraceptives and breast cancer that included a series of sensitivity analyses (42). These analyses revealed a small increase in the risk for breast cancer with the use of oral contraceptives that was independent of methodologic factors (design of the primary studies), study sample factors (age, ethnicity,

Table 10.3   *Continued*

←—Important Methodologic Characteristics—→				Outcomes			
Study Duration	Dropouts	Intervention Group	Comparison Group	Specific Outcome	Baseline Score ± SD	Follow-up Score ± SD	Change in Score (95% CI)
wk	*%*						
24	8	In-the-ear hearing aids	Waiting list	HHIE[†] Hearing aid Waiting list	48.7 ± 27.3 51.2 ± 29.1	14.7 ± 17.7 51.2 ± 28.0	34.0 (27.3–40.8)

and educational and reproductive background), context of the primary study (national setting), and drug factors (type and duration of drug therapy used). Subgroup analyses must be used with caution, however, because they are subject to many recognized limitations, including spurious associations that may be suggested by such "data dredging" (43). Finally, special types of meta-analysis that use individual patient data obtained from primary investigators may allow adjustment for heterogeneity and confounding by multiple factors (9, 44, 45). This approach is labor and resource intensive and, although potentially powerful, may not be possible in many circumstances.

Studies addressing similar questions often report different outcomes. For instance, controlled trials assessing the effect of interventions to reduce alcohol consumption may include biochemical markers, professional reports, or self-reports of abstinence as outcomes. In such circumstances, it may be possible to conduct separate meta-analyses for each key end point. As an alternative, standardized effect sizes or scale-free weighted mean differences can be used (the ratio of the difference between means in the treatment and control groups to the SD in the control group) (46). Standardized effect sizes help estimate whether an intervention has a consistent effect in a group of related outcomes. Limitations of the use of standardized effect sizes include the following: 1) All outcomes are given equal weight regardless of clinical significance, 2) misleading results may occur if unrelated outcomes are combined or if major differences in effects of the intervention on the different outcomes exist, and 3) bias may result if investigators have selectively reported their most positive results. Another approach is to derive a standardized definition for outcomes. For example, reviewers evaluating comprehensive geriatric assessment obtained unpublished information

from the original investigators on outcomes, such as functional status, that could be standardized across studies (47). A review of stroke unit trials used a standardized description of stroke services and a pre-established definition of disability that could be determined from several different disability scales (20). Similarly, standardized data were used in a review of adverse gastrointestinal effects associated with nonsteroidal anti-inflammatory drugs (48).

Conclusions

Reviewers interested in integrating many pieces of evidence face a kaleidoscope of research data that are fragmented by heterogeneity among study populations, exposures, diagnostic or intervention strategies, comparison groups, outcomes, study design, and quality. Although such heterogeneity may stimulate confidence by allowing assessment of general consistency and applicability, it may also increase uncertainty. Reviewers must therefore make judgments about the relevance of the heterogeneity, the legitimacy and relative uncertainty of particular pieces of evidence, the importance of missing pieces, the soundness of models for linking various pieces, and the appropriateness of conducting a quantitative summary. Integration of multiple pieces of disparate evidence is therefore a challenging and complex task that demands skill, humility, and skepticism. Initial steps involve recognition of distinction between direct and indirect evidence and the development of explicit models that break a complex problem into a series of smaller "subproblems" and hypothesize linkages among those subproblems. Focused systematic reviews for the important subproblems should be performed. Then, any of a variety of subjective or quantitative methods can be used to help integrate data into a unified whole. No single integrative approach is clearly superior, and some require specialized techniques.

None obviates uncertainty, all involve assumptions, and all ultimately underscore the role of careful judgment in integrating evidence.

Key Points To Remember

• Direct evidence relates an exposure, diagnostic strategy, or therapeutic intervention directly to the occurrence of a principal health outcome. Evidence is indirect if two or more bodies of evidence are required to relate the exposure, diagnostic strategy, or intervention to the principal health outcome.

• Explicit models provide analytic frameworks for viewing many pieces of evidence; they break a complex problem into a series of smaller subproblems and formally theorize linkages between those subproblems.

• Multiple factors, including heterogeneity of study populations, exposures or diagnostic or intervention strategies, comparison groups, outcomes, and study design and quality, contribute to the complexity of integrating direct and indirect evidence.

• Current methods for integrating heterogeneous evidence include a variety of evolving subjective and quantitative approaches.

Appendix

The concepts and examples outlined in this article are drawn from a wide variety of sources. We used the Cochrane Methodology Database for the core of information. We also used informal approaches, such as discussion with colleagues and workshops on complexity within systematic reviews that have been conducted at several international research symposia.

Acknowledgments: The authors thank Drs. Robert Fletcher and Brian Haynes for their critical reading of the manuscript. They also thank the clinical reviewer, Norman J. Wilder.

References

1. **Cook DJ, Mulrow CD, Haynes RB.** Systematic reviews: synthesis of best evidence for clinical decisions. Ann Intern Med. 1997;126:376-80.
2. **Hunt DL, McKibbon KA.** Locating and appraising systematic reviews. Ann Intern Med. 1997;126:532-8.
3. **McQuay HJ, Moore A.** Using numerical results from systematic reviews in clinical practice. Ann Intern Med. 1997;126:712-20.
4. **Badgett RG, O'Keefe M, Henderson MC.** Using systematic reviews in clinical education. Ann Intern Med. 1997;126:886-91.
5. **Bero LA, Jadad AR.** How consumers and policy-makers can use systematic reviews for decision making. Ann Intern Med. 1997;127:37-42.
6. **Cook DJ, Greengold NL, Ellrodt AG, Weingarten SR.** The relation between systematic reviews in practice guidelines. Ann Intern Med. 1997;127:210-6.
7. **Counsell C.** Formulating questions and locating primary studies for inclusion in systematic reviews. Ann Intern Med. 1997;127:380-7.
8. **Meade MO, Richardson WS.** Selecting and appraising studies for a systematic review. Ann Intern Med. 1997;127:531-7.
9. **Lau J, Ioannidis JP, Schmid CH.** Quantitative synthesis in systematic reviews. Ann Intern Med. 1997;127:820-6.
10. **Cooper HM.** The analysis and interpretation stage. In: The Integrative Research Review: A Systematic Approach. Beverly Hills, CA: Sage; 1984:79-113.
11. **Kerlinger FN.** Foundations of Behavioral Research. 2d ed. New York: Holt, Rinehart, and Winston; 1973.
12. **Eddy DM, Hasselblad V, Shachter R.** Meta-Analysis by the Confidence Profile Method: The Statistical Synthesis of Evidence. San Diego: Academic Pr; 1992.
13. **Fleming TR, DeMets DL.** Surrogate end points in clinical trials: are we being misled? Ann Intern Med. 1996;125:605-13.
14. **Collins R, Peto R, MacMahon S, Hebert P, Fiebach NH, Eberlein KA, et al.** Blood pressure, stroke, and coronary heart disease. Part 2, Short-term reductions in blood pressure: overview of randomised drug trials in their epidemiological context. Lancet. 1990;335:827-38.
15. **Shepherd J, Cobbe SM, Ford I, Isles CG, Lorimer AR, MacFarlane PW, et al.** Prevention of coronary heart disease with pravastatin in men with hypercholesterolemia. West of Scotland Coronary Prevention Study Group. N Engl J Med. 1995;333:1301-7.
16. **Sacks FM, Pfeffer MA, Moye LA, Rouleau JL, Rutherford JD, Cole TG, et al.** The effect of pravastatin on coronary events after myocardial infarction in patients with average cholesterol levels. Cholesterol and Recurrent Events Trial Investigators. N Engl J Med. 1996;335:1001-9.
17. Randomised trial of cholesterol lowering in 4444 patients with coronary heart disease: the

Scandinavian Simvastatin Survival Study (4S). Lancet. 1994;344:1383-9.

18. **Wolff SH.** Manual for Clinical Practice Guideline Development. Rockville, MD: Agency for Health Care Policy and Research; 1991. AHCPR publication no. 91-0007.

19. **Battista RN, Fletcher SW.** Making recommendations on preventive practices: methodological issues. Am J Prev Med. 1988;4(4 Suppl):53-67.

20. **Stroke Unit Trialists' Collaboration.** A systematic review of specialist multidisciplinary (stroke unit) care for stroke inpatients. In: Warlow C, Van Gijn J, Sandercock P, eds. Stroke Module of the Cochrane Database of Systematic Reviews. London: BMJ Publishing Group; 1995.

21. **Davis DA, Thomson MA, Oxman AD, Haynes RB.** Changing physician performance. A systematic review of the effect of continuing medical education strategies. JAMA. 1995;274:700-5.

22. **Grimshaw JM, Freemantle N, Langhorne P, Song F.** Complexity and Systematic Reviews. Report to the U.S. Congress of Technology Assessment. Washington, DC: Office of Technology Assessment; 1995.

23. **Mulrow CD, Lichtenstein MJ.** Screening for hearing impairment in the elderly: rationale and strategy. J Gen Intern Med. 1991;6:249-58.

24. **Cadman D, Chambers L, Feldman W, Sackett D.** Assessing the effectiveness of community screening programs. JAMA. 1984;251:1580-5.

25. **Bradford-Hill A.** The environment and disease: association or causation? Proc Roy Soc Med. 1965;58:295-300.

26. **Huff J.** A historical perspective on the classification developed and used for chemical carcinogens by the National Toxicology Program during 1983-1992. Scand J Work Environ Health. 1992;18(Suppl 1):74-82.

27. **Koes BW, Bouter LM, Beckerman H, van der Heijden GJ, Knipschild PG.** Physiotherapy exercises and back pain: a blinded review. Br Med J. 1991;302:1572-6.

28. **Canadian Task Force on the Periodic Health Examination.** The periodic health examination. Can Med Assoc J. 1979;121:1193-254.

29. **Cook DJ, Guyatt GH, Laupacis A, Sackett DL, Goldberg RJ.** Clinical recommendations using levels of evidence for antithrombotic agents. Chest. 1995;108:227-305.

30. Acute Pain Management: Operative or Medical Procedures and Trauma. Rockville, MD: U.S. Department of Health and Human Services, Public Health Service, Agency for Health Care Policy and Research; 1992. AHCPR no. 92-00038.

31. **Carruthers SG, Larochelle P, Haynes RB, Petrasovits A, Schiffrin EL.** Canadian Hypertension Society Consensus Conference: 1. Introduction. Can Med Assoc J. 1993;149:289-93.

32. **Guyatt GH, Sackett DL, Sinclair JC, Hayward R, Cook DJ, Cook RJ, et al.** Users' guides to the medical literature. IX. A method for grading health care recommendations. Evidence-Based Medicine Working Group. JAMA. 1995;274:1800-4.

33. **Light RJ, Pillemer DB.** Summing Up: The Science of Reviewing Research. Cambridge, MA: Harvard Univ Pr; 1984.

34. **Eddy DM.** Comparing benefits and harms: the balance sheet. JAMA. 1990;263:2493-505.

35. **U.S. Preventive Services Task Force.** Guide to Clinical Preventive Services. 2d ed. Baltimore: Williams & Wilkins; 1996.

36. **Weinstein MC, Fineberg HV, Elstein AS, Frazier HS, Neuhauser D, Neutra RR, et al.** Clinical Decision Analysis. Philadelphia: WB Saunders; 1980.

37. **Berger J.** Statistical Decision Theory and Bayesian Analysis. New York: Springer-Verlag; 1985.

38. **Gold MR, Siegel JE, Russell LB, Weinstein MC, eds.** Cost-Effectiveness in Health and Medicine. New York: Oxford Univ Pr; 1996.

39. **Tijms HC.** Stochastic modelling and analysis: a computational approach. Chichester, United Kingdom: J Wiley; 1986.

40. **Ross SM.** Introduction to Probability Models. 3d ed. Berkeley, CA: Academic Pr; 1985.

41. **Gotzsche PC.** Methodology and overt and hidden bias in reports of 196 double-blind trials of nonsteroidal antiinflammatory drugs in rheumatoid arthritis. Control Clin Trials. 1989;10:31-56.

42. **Collaborative Group on Hormonal Factors in Breast Cancer.** Breast cancer and hormonal contraceptives: collaborative reanalysis of individual data on 53 297 women with breast cancer and 100 239 women without breast cancer from 54 epidemiological studies. Lancet. 1996;347:1713-27.

43. **Oxman AD, Guyatt GH.** A consumer's guide to subgroup analyses. Ann Intern Med. 1992;116:78-84.

44. **Stewart LA, Clarke MJ.** Practical methodology of meta-analyses (overviews) using updated individual patient data. Cochrane Working Group. Stat Med. 1995;14:2057-79.

45. **Antiplatelet Trialists' Collaboration.** Collaborative overview of randomised trials of antiplatelet treatment-III: Reduction in venous thrombosis and pulmonary embolism by antiplatelet prophylaxis among surgical and medical patients. BMJ. 1994;308:235-46.

46. **Berkey CS, Anderson JJ, Hoaglin DC.** Multiple-outcome meta-analysis of clinical trials. Stat Med. 1996;14:537-57.

47. **Stuck AE, Siu AL, Wieland GD, Adams J, Rubenstein LZ.** Comprehensive geriatric assessment: a meta-analysis of controlled trials. Lancet. 1993;342:1032-6.

48. **Henry D, Lim LL, Garcia Rodriguez LA, Gutthann SP, Carson JL, Griffin SM, et al.** Variability in risk of gastrointestinal complications with individual non-steroidal and anti-inflammatory drugs: results of a collaborative meta-analysis. BMJ. 1996;312:1563-6.

Index